Contents

EPILEPSY

The Essential Guide by Louise Bolotin

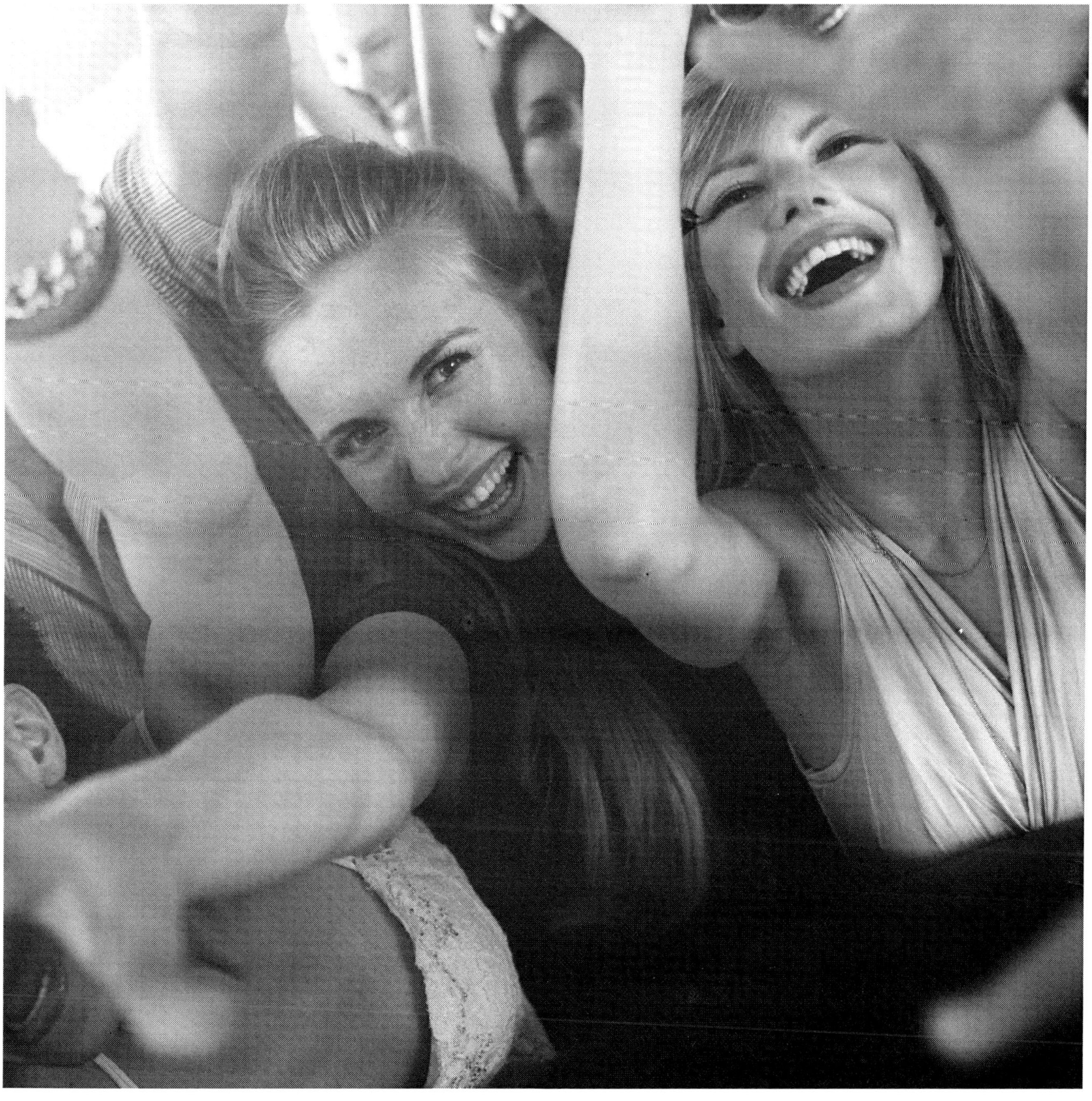

First published in Great Britain in 2009 by
Need2Know
Remus House
Coltsfoot Drive
Peterborough
PE2 9BF
Telephone 01733 898103
Fax 01733 313524
www.need2knowbooks.co.uk
Large Print Edition 2011.

Need2Know is an imprint of Bonacia Ltd.
www.need2knowbooks.co.uk

SB ISBN 978-1-86144-152-2

Introduction

Every second of every day, our bodies transmit electrical signals through our nerves. These electric signals contain important information to ensure that the body carries out the brain's instructions. For example, you want to read a book so your brain tells your hand to pick up the book and open it, and it all happens so quickly that your hand has already opened the book by the time you are even conscious that you made the decision to read it.

Epilepsy causes problems with the brain's electrical activity – it disrupts those signals and stops both brain and body working properly for brief periods of time. Imagine that a fuse blows in the fuse box at your house and causes a power cut. The lights suddenly go out and you are sitting in the dark. The TV no longer works, the phone's down too and even your doorbell is not working. Worse, your computer has crashed while you were in the middle of doing something. Groping around in the dark, you finally manage to reset the fuses. The lights come back on and your TV powers up again. Your computer reboots itself but it takes a while to open all the programs again. The file you were working on has to be rescued from the last saved version and some data is missing.

This is how it can feel to have an epileptic seizure and then come round from it. Like that crashed computer, the brain needs a little time to reboot afterwards and some data may be lost, such as your memory of exactly what you were doing before the seizure started.

Being diagnosed with epilepsy can be frightening for many people as this very misunderstood condition carries much stigma and has many myths attached to it. Yet epilepsy is the commonest neurological disorder – one in 133 people have it and one in 20 people will have at least one seizure in their lifetime. The vast majority – 70% – of people with epilepsy gain good or total control over their seizures on the right medication and it's possible to live a normal life after diagnosis, albeit with some minor restrictions.

When people think of epilepsy, they imagine the classic scenario of someone writhing unconscious on the ground and frothing at the mouth. While this may be true for some people (although any froth is more likely to be a dribble of saliva), there are in fact many types of seizure, all very different from each other. Some people may have only one kind of seizure, others could have several. Epilepsy is a very individual condition, meaning that no two people diagnosed with it are likely to have the same experience or symptoms or be treated with the same medication.

There is no doubt that for some people with epilepsy it can be debilitating. Poorly controlled seizures increase the risk of injuries and other complications, so finding the right medication at the right dosage is usually the first priority. Children who have epilepsy often have other problems too, particularly if diagnosed very young. They may have learning difficulties, for example, or other physical disabilities. Older people have to face other issues such as maintaining independence. And for everyone in between there are many questions that need answering: Can I work? Should I tell my boss? Will I be able to have children? Is it okay to drink alcohol? Will I ever be able to drive again? Can I play football? Can I go swimming?

This book, as the title suggests, aims to provide essential guidance for you if you have just been diagnosed with epilepsy and want support. It can also be used by your family, friends, teachers or colleagues if they want to understand the condition and be able to offer you practical and emotional help.

Neurology services in the UK are very stretched – there is a national shortage of neurologists who specialise in epilepsy and although some departments have specialist epilepsy nurses on hand to answer questions, it's a lottery as to whether you'll have access to one. In these circumstances, it can be hard to have your questions answered fully.

Epilepsy – The Essential Guide will take you through all the aspects of living with epilepsy. Diagnosis and the different types of seizure are explained, as well as providing you with all the practical information you need to live your life as normally as possible after diagnosis: from why showers are better than baths to when you should ring for an ambulance.

Throughout the chapters you will find references to helpful resources – further information can be found in the help list at the back of the book. There is also a glossary at the very end to explain some of the most common medical terms used in epilepsy care.

Disclaimer

This book is only for general information about epilepsy and the author advises that she does not claim medical qualifications. It is not intended to replace medical advice, although it can be used alongside it. Anyone who has epilepsy or suspects they could have it should seek medical advice from a healthcare professional such as a GP or NHS drop-in surgery.

Epilepsy – the Basics

What is epilepsy?

Epilepsy is a neurological disorder characterised by seizures, or fits, as a result of disruption to the brain's electrical impulses. It can take a number of different forms.

As seizures may be a symptom of other medical problems (for example, diabetes, alcoholism or drug abuse), epilepsy is only usually considered after at least two seizures have occurred. There is no cure for epilepsy but it is treatable – mainly with medication, sometimes with surgery.

What causes epilepsy?

Epilepsy can be caused by a number of different factors. For roughly four in 10 people, there will be a specific cause such as head injury, genetic inheritance, brain damage caused by a stroke, an illness such as meningitis or a difficult birth, or some other physical cause such as a brain tumour. Where the cause is known, this is called symptomatic epilepsy.

Epilepsy can be caused by a number of different factors. For roughly four in 10 people, there will be a specific structural cause such as head injury, brain damage caused by a stroke, an illness such as meningitis or a difficult birth, or some other physical cause such as a brain tumour. Where the cause is known, this is called symptomatic epilepsy. Where the cause is an inherited genetic disorder or the result of a genetic defect, this is known as idiopathic epilepsy.

Cryptogenic epilepsy is the term used where a known cause for epilepsy is suspected but cannot be proven. For the other 60% who have epilepsy, the cause is never known.

Diagnosis

Diagnosing epilepsy is not an exact science. Your GP is likely to be the first doctor you see if you are experiencing symptoms that could indicate you have epilepsy. Doctors have an unwritten rule of thumb that 'everyone is allowed one seizure', as one in 20 people will have a seizure of some kind at some point in their life. Only if you have had two or more seizures is your GP likely to refer you to a neurologist, ideally one who specialises in epilepsy, to carry out any tests and reach a diagnosis.

There is no one special test that gives a definitive diagnosis, although some tests can give strong pointers. The most common tests are an EEG and a brain scan of some sort (either a CT scan or an MRI scan). Doctors also take into account witness descriptions (if someone has seen you have a seizure) as these can help confirm diagnosis. If you have a friend or relative who has witnessed you having a seizure, ask them to accompany you when you see the specialist as any descriptions they can provide can be invaluable. All this information will be looked at as a whole to confirm a diagnosis, along with the specialist's own clinical expertise.

The EEG test

You are most likely to have an EEG (electroencephalogram). This measures and records the patterns of electrical activity in the brain. Epilepsy usually produces specific unusual patterns, so an EEG can often pinpoint a diagnosis. However, these patterns do not occur all the time, so the EEG only captures a snapshot of the electrical patterns at the time of the test. Consequently, it may be necessary to repeat the test at a later date.

The EEG takes around 30 minutes. You wear a special cap on your head that has holes in it. The nurse will squirt some conductor gel through the holes then attach 20 to 30 electrodes to your head. It can be slightly uncomfortable but is not painful or dangerous. Once the cap is on and you have been wired up, you will be asked to lie down and your brain activity will start to get recorded. During the recording you will be asked to open and close your eyes and to breathe deeply then shallowly. After the test, the nurse should offer you the opportunity to wash your hair. You may want to take your own shampoo and conditioner with you – the conductor gel can be sticky but washes out with a thorough shampooing. The EEG test results will be analysed and sent to your GP or consultant.

Brain scans

Sometimes it is not possible for a strong diagnosis through an EEG, even if it has been done more than once. If the suspected cause of epilepsy is a head injury, a tumour or some other identifiable physical cause, you may have a CT (computed tomography) scan or an MRI (magnetic resonance imaging) scan.

The CT scan is a method of creating a three-dimensional image of the brain using two-dimensional x-rays. It is completely painless – you lie on a bed and the scanner takes digital x-ray pictures in slices of your brain. The test usually takes 10 to 30 minutes.

An MRI scan is similar to a CT scan but more sophisticated. The scanner uses a magnetic field to create images of the brain and typically takes between 20 to 30 minutes. It can be uncomfortable as you lie completely still on a bed that is fed into a narrow scanner tube, and the magnets can be very noisy while they scan you. For these reasons, it is not suitable if you suffer from claustrophobia.

Once tests have been carried out, your doctor will piece together all the information including any descriptions of seizures that were witnessed. If epilepsy is confirmed, treatment options will be discussed with you.

Coming to terms with diagnosis

Even when you know you might have epilepsy, the diagnosis can still be a shock. This confirmation is likely to have an immediate and long-term impact on your life and can take time to come to terms with, especially as you may have to deal with some immediate restrictions on your lifestyle.

It is a good idea to take a friend or relative with you when you are called to discuss your test results. This is because you may find the diagnosis hard to take in at first and you might not remember everything the doctor tells you. Having someone with you means they are more likely to remember what you are told. You may also want to take a pen and paper to write things down. If you suspect in advance that you will be diagnosed with epilepsy, you could even prepare a list of questions to ask (see chapter 4 for ideas).

Give yourself time to accept the diagnosis before making any lifestyle decisions and ask your doctor if they can provide you with written information about living with epilepsy. If you have seen a neurologist, there may be an epilepsy nurse attached to the clinic who can talk through any questions you have and help you think through some of the decisions you will need to consider (see chapter 3). If you have been diagnosed by your GP, you might want to ask for a referral to a neurologist for specialist care. Whatever options you are offered, don't be afraid of asking for an appointment with an appropriate specialist to talk through all the issues and concerns you have.

Types of epilepsy

The brain is a massively complex organ but consists, very simply, of two main sections – the cortex and the cerebellum. These are further divided into lobes. The cortex, which is responsible for functions such as memory, thought, language, movement and awareness, contains the frontal, parietal, occipital and temporal lobes. It is within one of these four lobes that a seizure will start, and they also determine what symptoms you may display during the seizure. Note that a seizure may start in more than one lobe at the same time and that a generalised seizure will affect all four lobes of the brain.

- Temporal lobes – these lobes control sensory functions such as speech, smell, taste and hearing, as well as emotions and memory.
- Frontal lobes – these are responsible for movement, language, social and sexual behaviour, our personality, emotions and memory.
- Parietal lobes – these control spatial awareness and visual processing, as well as sensory information from other parts of the body.
- Occipital lobes – these lobes control our vision.

There are around 50 different types of seizure or seizure syndromes. This book will only look at the most common ones and the chapter on children will briefly cover some syndromes specific to them.

Partial seizures

Partial seizures are sometimes called focal seizures and can be simple or complex. Partials start in one of the lobes but do not spread to the rest of the brain, unless they evolve into a secondary generalised seizure (see below). During a simple partial you remain conscious and fully aware of everything happening around you. However, you will not be able to stop what is happening to you – you may find, for example, that you cannot speak during the seizure or that you cannot control your limbs.

In a complex partial your consciousness can be affected briefly and you may be unaware of what is happening to you or what you are doing. When you return to consciousness you will probably have little memory of what has happened and what you do remember may be hazy.

Partial seizures in the temporal lobe

Because the temporal lobes control sensory functions, partial seizures can involve a wide range of symptoms that can be distressing to experience.

During a simple partial, you may:

- Start sweating or flushing, or turn pale.
- Feel as if your stomach is churning.
- Experience visual or auditory disturbances such as hallucinations or distortions of what you can see or hear.
- Taste or smell things that don't exist.
- Have false or real 'flashbacks' to memories, or sensations of *déjà vu.*
- Experience intense emotions such as fear, elation, melancholy or panic. You might also feel detached from your surroundings

During a complex partial, you may:

- Make repetitive physical movements such as scratching, swallowing, chewing or smacking your lips.
- Undo buttons or zips on your clothes or even start undressing yourself.
- Wander off – you may come round in a different room or outside, with no recollection of how you got there.

Partial seizures in the frontal lobe

As with the temporal lobe, partials in the frontal lobe can produce some distressing actions which are physical rather than emotional.

Typical symptoms include:

- Stiffness in your arms or fingers, with possible jerking or thrashing.
- Strange body movements such as 'cycling' or kicking your legs.
- Difficulty making people understand what you are saying.
- Acting out sexual feelings or behaviour which may or may not be overt.
- Shouting, crying or swearing.
- Incontinence of the bladder or bowel.

Frontal lobe symptoms can appear bizarre to onlookers. For this reason, frontal lobe seizures can sometimes be misdiagnosed by a GP as psychiatric or other behavioural problems or neurological disorders such as Tourette's syndrome.

Partial seizures in the parietal lobe

Partials in the parietal lobes produce strange bodily sensations known as sensory seizures.

Typical symptoms include:

- Tingling or warmness, often only down one side of the body.

- Numbness in parts of the body.
- Feeling that your limbs are bigger or smaller than they really are.

Partial seizures in the occipital lobe

Partials in the occipital lobes result in visual disturbances.

Typical symptoms include:

- Flashing lights or balls of light which may or may not be coloured.
- Hallucinations.
- Temporary loss of vision.

Both simple and complex partials usually last anywhere from around 10–15 seconds to a minute or so. During these types of seizure, anyone who tries to talk to you may not understand what you are experiencing and it is possible they could react badly towards you. When you return to full consciousness afterwards, you may feel confused for a while. You could also develop a strong headache, feel tired and need a nap.

Todd's paralysis (Todd's paresis)

Sometimes after a partial seizure you may find that part of your body is paralysed. This is known as Todd's paralysis – it is quite rare and is also temporary. The paralysis might wear off after a few minutes or it may take several hours to go completely. It should not result in any harm but is often frustrating to experience.

Auras

Sometimes a simple partial seizure can develop into a generalised seizure (see the next page). When this happens it is called an aura or warning because you will often be aware that you are going to have a bigger seizure. This simple partial seizure gives you enough time to make yourself safe before you fall unconscious.

Generalised seizures

Seizures that affect the whole brain from the very start are called generalised seizures. A secondary generalised seizure is one that starts in one part of the brain (a partial seizure) and then spreads to all other areas. In either case, you will experience loss of consciousness. There are several distinct types of generalised seizure.

Absence seizures

Absences (sometimes called petit mal) mainly affect children, although adults can also experience them. Absences can occur very frequently – many times per day is not unusual. During an absence you may appear to others as if you are daydreaming or blank-faced and staring, but the absence may be so short that no one notices. In fact, you will have fallen briefly unconscious – typically for 10-15 seconds, absences lasting 20-30 seconds are considered abnormal – and will be unaware of your surroundings. You will not fall to the ground, have convulsions or jerk your limbs. When you return to consciousness it is likely you will not be aware that you had briefly switched off.

Children who have absence seizures can be affected developmentally – see chapter 7 for further information.

Tonic and atonic seizures

These two seizure types are very similar – in both types there is usually no warning. A typical seizure will last 15-30 seconds and recovery will be very fast. During a tonic seizure your muscles suddenly become very stiff and you may fall backwards if you are standing. Tonic seizures are common during sleep, if you have them. In an atonic seizure, sometimes called a drop attack, your muscles will suddenly become very floppy and you will fall down, usually forwards.

Because of the very high risk of falling, you also have a high risk of injury, particularly to the head. If you have frequent seizures of this type, you might want to consider buying a protective helmet (see help list).

Myoclonic seizures

The term 'myoclonic' means 'muscle jerk'. A myoclonic seizure means that one or more limbs jerk and you will fall unconscious, but so briefly that it is barely noticeable.

Myoclonic seizures tend to be very brief but it's possible to experience a cluster of them in a short space of time. The jerking mostly affects the arms or head but can affect the legs, possibly causing you to fall over.

This type of seizure is commonest soon after waking and they mostly occur in conjunction with other seizure types, such as tonic-clonic seizures (see below).

Myoclonic jerks can result in injuries, not just from falling but from tipping hot drinks over yourself or bashing your limbs against furniture.

Tonic-clonic seizures

The tonic-clonic seizure, occasionally called grand mal, is the classic convulsive seizure most people recognise as epilepsy (where you fall unconscious and thrash around). It is also the type of seizure most likely to follow an aura.

There are two phases that follow each other in quick succession. In the tonic phase your muscles go rigid and, if you are standing or even seated, you will fall to the floor. As the muscles tighten, air is forced out of your lungs, causing an involuntary cry. The loss of air in the lungs is temporary but to onlookers you may appear to go blue in the face and your breathing may be erratic and noisy. You may also bite the insides of your cheeks or tongue.

In the clonic phase your muscles will contract and relax rapidly, causing your limbs to jerk. You may become incontinent. You may also appear to froth at the mouth, but in reality it's likely to be a dribble of saliva with a few air bubbles blown through your lips. Both phases together typically last between one and five minutes, with two minutes being around average.

Recovery from a tonic-clonic is known as the post-ictal phase. Recovery times vary a lot – you are likely to return to consciousness fairly quickly, but it could take 30 minutes or so before you are fully aware you have had a seizure. A very severe headache may start within an hour of return to consciousness – you can treat this with some paracetamol or other painkiller. Some people occasionally feel nauseous or vomit during recovery. You will probably feel very tired and want to sleep – go to bed if you can and sleep for as long as you feel you need to. Later, your body might ache from the muscle contractions – a hot shower or light exercise such as a walk may help and anti-inflammatory painkillers such as ibuprofen can also ease stiffness. Do not be surprised if full recovery takes up to 24 hours.

Nocturnal seizures

It is possible to have seizures while you are asleep. Some people only ever have seizures during the night, but others can experience them both awake and sleeping. The commonest type of nocturnal seizure is the tonic-clonic, but partial seizures are also possible. Often you may only be aware that you have had a sleep seizure when you wake up and realise you have a post-seizure headache and stiff muscles.

The process of diagnosis is similar to that for waking seizures. You will probably have an EEG test. If this is inconclusive, it may be repeated as a sleep-deprivation test – you will be asked to stay up all night (or as long as possible) before having the EEG first thing in the morning. Alternatively, you could be asked to have an overnight EEG test at the hospital or even a 24-hour one. If you have a partner or family member who has witnessed a nocturnal seizure, they will be asked to describe it to help confirm diagnosis.

As with waking seizures, you are most likely to be prescribed medication to control your nocturnal seizures. It is also important to have a good bedtime routine and a regular amount of sleep as overtiredness can trigger night seizures.

Your safety needs to be considered as there is a risk you may fall out of bed during a seizure. Sleeping in a low bed will minimise the drop and a deep-pile rug or carpet will help cushion your landing. Try and avoid synthetic fibres in any floor coverings as they may cause friction burns, and choose only bedside furniture, like tables, with rounded edges to reduce the risk of head wounds. If you share your home with others, you may find having a bed alarm is useful to alert them to come to your assistance.

Photo-sensitive epilepsy

Around 5% of people with epilepsy are photo-sensitive, which means their seizures are triggered by flashing lights or similar effects such as geometric patterns or sunlight through trees. Sometimes photo-sensitivity is detected during the EGG test, but many people only discover this tendency when a seizure is actually triggered. It is commonest among people under the age of 20 and usually induces a tonic-clonic seizure.

The key to photo-sensitivity is the rate or frequency of any flashing. If you are photo-sensitive, you are likely to react to a rate of three to 30 flickers per second (the flash rate is called hertz). Triggers can include strobe lights in night-clubs, video games, old TV sets that flicker, broken fluorescent striplights and rippling sunlight. The risk of a seizure increases if you are tired, stressed or overexcited.

If you have a modern computer screen or TV set, you are unlikely to be affected because they don't flicker. Also, broadcasters are restricted in what they can show but must give a warning if any TV programme contains flashing within the risk range of the hertz cycle.

You can cut your risk of having a seizure by using the TV or computer in a well-lit room, not sitting too close to the screen, taking regular screen breaks and wearing tinted glasses or sunglasses when outside in sunny conditions.

Myths about epilepsy

People with epilepsy swallow their tongues

It is a popular belief that someone having a seizure may swallow their tongue and die and that this can be prevented by inserting a spoon in the mouth. It is physically impossible to swallow the tongue, although it may briefly flop onto the back of the throat, impeding breathing. You are more likely to bite your tongue or inner cheeks during a seizure – these types of injury usually heal quickly without medical treatment and only require some antiseptic mouthwash to help stop any bleeding or infection.

People with epilepsy are possessed

Epilepsy is a neurological condition, meaning the brain has a physical disorder. Some non-European cultures still believe that someone having a convulsive seizure must be possessed by the devil. This link with religious belief is not unusual – St Paul's vision on the road to Damascus is now thought by many specialists to fit the description of temporal lobe epilepsy. Shamanistic religions believe their shaman gains wisdom or insights when they go into a trance or shake, yet they may simply be experiencing an epileptic seizure.

People with epilepsy can't look at flashing lights

This is only partly true. Around 5% of people who have epilepsy react to flashing lights or strobing (see the section on photosensitive epilepsy), but for most people this is not a problem at all.

Summing Up

Epilepsy is a neurological condition that affects those who have it on a very individual basis. You are likely to have one or more tests if your doctor suspects you have epilepsy. However, diagnosis cannot be determined by tests alone and other factors will be taken into account. If you have been diagnosed, ask your doctor what type of epilepsy you have, as there are many different kinds, and how it may affect you.

First Aid and Mortality Issues

Whether you have epilepsy yourself or are a friend, relative or carer of someone who has it, it is wise to familiarise yourself with certain important issues. There are standard first aid procedures for someone having a convulsive seizure and it is important not only to know what to do but also to know what not to do. Unfortunately, there is a risk of dying from an epileptic seizure but the risk is slight overall. However, being aware of the possibility and knowing how to reduce your risk could save your life (or a friend or relative's).

First aid

Seeing someone have a full-blown convulsive (tonic-clonic) seizure can be scary, but there is no need to panic and it is rare to need to call for medical assistance. Most seizures last only a short time (up to five minutes) and stop without any special treatment. Injuries can occur but most people do not come to any harm in a seizure and do not usually need to go to hospital or see a doctor. When a person has a convulsive seizure it is possible that their regular breathing pattern will be affected and they may go blue. Although this can be frightening to witness, it does not usually mean it is a medical emergency.

During the seizure:

- Let the seizure run its course and stay calm.
- Do not try and restrain the person as this could cause injuries.
- Note the time and length of the seizure.
- Prevent other people from crowding round.
- Put soft cushioning under the person's head to prevent injury. Improvise if necessary – you can roll up your jacket, for example.

- Only move them if they are in danger, for example from tumbling down stairs. Move things like items of furniture away if there is a risk of injury.
- Never, ever attempt to put anything in the person's mouth. There is no danger of swallowing the tongue and the teeth or jaw can easily be broken. You are also at risk of having your own fingers bitten!

When the seizure has stopped:

- If you can, roll the person onto their side in the recovery position.
- Wipe away any excess saliva. If breathing seems laboured, check there is nothing blocking the throat, such as dentures or food.
- Do what you can to reduce any embarrassment. If the person has wet themselves, try to deal with this privately.
- Stay with the person, giving reassurance, until they have fully recovered. This could take 30 minutes or longer. Just talk gently to them and repeat that they've had a seizure until they fully understand this. Do not offer them a drink unless you are sure they are fully recovered. Expect them to want a long sleep after they have returned to full consciousness.

When to call for help

Call the paramedics immediately if any of the following apply:

- The person has injured themselves badly in a seizure. Head injuries in particular should always be checked out by a qualified medic.
- The person has trouble breathing after a seizure.
- One seizure immediately follows another with no recovery in between.
- The seizure continues for longer than is usual for that person.
- The seizure is still on-going after five minutes when it is not known how long they usually last for that person.

- It is the person's first seizure.

Where seizures continue with no break or no recovery period in between, calling the paramedics could save a life. This condition is called status (see below) and, although rare, can result in death or severe brain damage, so call an ambulance immediately and stay with them until help arrives.

Status

Status epilepticus, usually called status, is a rare condition that can be life-threatening. When you are diagnosed, you may not be told about status but it is important to be aware of it.

Usually each seizure you have will last around the same amount of time. How long this is depends on what is typical for you. It may be 30 seconds or it could be up to five minutes. Normally, your seizure will come to a natural end and then you will go into your recovery period which could be 30 minutes or longer.

Sometimes, though, your seizure may not stop or you may have one or more seizures after the first one without a recovery period in between. When a seizure lasts like this for 30 minutes or longer, you are in status.

Whatever type of seizures you have, particularly tonic-clonic, status can occur. This is a medical emergency as you could suffer brain damage or even die. It is vital that someone calls an ambulance before 30 minutes has passed. Usually it will be obvious after 10 minutes or so if the seizures are on-going and show no sign of stopping. See the previous section on first aid for information on when to call for an ambulance.

Some people who regularly go into status can be prescribed emergency medication, usually rectal diazepam or buccal midazolam, to stop the seizures. Whoever administers these drugs – whether a paramedic or carer – must have training on how to give them correctly. Your carer should also have a written protocol (treatment plan) to follow if you go into status.

SUDEP

What is SUDEP?

Sudden unexpected death in epilepsy (SUDEP) is a very rare condition where someone who has epilepsy dies suddenly and there is no obvious cause of death. Sadly, it is also rare for doctors to tell you about SUDEP when you are diagnosed, but every year bewildered family and friends of someone who has died from SUDEP have to deal with the fact that they had no idea their loved one might be at risk of death. It is important to be aware of SUDEP and have an understanding of what it is while also remembering to keep a sense of perspective about the risks.

Around 500 to 600 people die from SUDEP annually in the UK out of approximately 450,000 people who have epilepsy. Very little is known about the causes of SUDEP. Researchers know that people who die from SUDEP usually die during or after a seizure, and usually while asleep, but it is not really understood why this can happen. Studies seem to point to the person's breathing or heart stopping but the research has yet to uncover anything more concrete.

Your risk level

Your personal risk level will depend entirely on what type of epilepsy you have, how it affects you and how well controlled your seizures are. The risk of SUDEP rises if you have nocturnal seizures, your seizures are poorly controlled, you do not take your medication properly or you have had your medication changed abruptly or frequently. If you are a young adult male or have learning disabilities, the risk is also higher but it is not properly understood why.

Reducing your risk

The easiest and most important way to reduce your risk is to take your medication as prescribed. Never stop taking your medication without the approval of your doctor as abrupt withdrawal from anti-epileptic drugs (AEDs) can actually trigger seizures.

It goes without saying that controlling your alcohol intake and not taking recreational drugs will also reduce your risk of SUDEP. Good quality sleep is also known to reduce the likelihood of having a seizure. See chapter 4 for information on alcohol, drugs and sleep.

If you are a friend or relative of someone who has epilepsy, you can play an active role in reducing their risk of dying from SUDEP. Familiarise yourself with the first aid procedures for seizures. If they appear to stop breathing after a seizure, being able to give simple mouth-to-mouth resuscitation (CPR or cardiopulmonary resuscitation) can help to kickstart breathing again while you call for medical assistance. When the seizure ends, put them in the recovery position and stay with them until they have regained full consciousness and are aware of their surroundings. This can take up to 30 minutes.

If you still have worries about SUDEP, talk them over with your doctor or an epilepsy nurse if you have access to one. They can help you assess your own level of risk and suggest ways to reduce it. The charity Epilepsy Bereaved can also provide detailed advice on the risks of SUDEP, including information over the telephone (see help list for details).

Summing Up

It's a good idea to familiarise yourself with first aid procedures for epileptic seizures – you may want to let your friends or relatives know how they can help if you have a seizure in their presence.
It can also be very difficult to face the fact that your risk of dying increases if you have epilepsy, especially if you have just been diagnosed and are already trying to come to terms with living with a long-term health condition. However, there is a strong argument for being aware of your mortality risk as there are steps you can take to reduce it. As with many medical conditions, knowledge can give you greater control of your health.

Treatments

After you have been diagnosed with epilepsy, it is very likely you will be prescribed treatment of some sort. In the first instance this is likely to be medication. More invasive options, such as surgery, are usually only considered if drug therapy proves unworkable.

The following information is only a brief guide to treatments. You are advised to seek medical advice from a qualified specialist.

NICE guidelines for diagnosis and treatment

The National Institute for Clinical Excellence (NICE), which sets standards for patient care in the NHS, issued clinical practice guidelines in 2004 on the diagnosis and management of epilepsy for both adults and children in England and Wales (SIGN in Scotland). The guidelines offer clear recommendations on how people with epilepsy are offered access to specialists and treatments.

The recommendations are lengthy but the main points include the following:

- Where a diagnosis of epilepsy is a possibility, you should be seen within two weeks by a specialist who has expertise in epilepsy to ensure accurate diagnosis and appropriate treatment.
- You should be offered fast-track access to appropriate diagnostic procedures such as MRI scans and EEG tests.
- You should be offered an individualised care plan upon diagnosis, as well as a structured review of this care plan at least once a year.
- If you have poorly controlled seizures, or have not had a clear diagnosis, you should be referred to a specialist tertiary service (see glossary) as soon as possible to ensure accurate diagnosis and optimal treatment and to reduce the risk of SUDEP.

- You have the right to be at the centre of all decisions on treating and managing your epilepsy.
- You have the right to be issued with non-generic prescription medication in order to maintain control over your seizures.
- You have the right to be provided with information about your epilepsy. This also applies to your carer, if you have one. You are also entitled to specialist advice if you are a woman of child-bearing age who may want to start a family.
- Children and adults who have both epilepsy and learning disabilities have the right to equality of access to NHS epilepsy services.

Epilepsy care within the NHS

Epilepsy care varies wildly across the NHS. Some of this is down to differences in interpretation of NHS rules and NICE guidelines among the various Primary Care Trusts (PCTs) who manage NHS care at regional level. Other reasons include the availability of specialist care. Most hospitals have a neurology clinic but these services are notoriously stretched and not all neurologists have a strong knowledge of epilepsy, having chosen to specialise in other areas.

It is possible that you might be referred to a neurologist whose knowledge of epilepsy amounts to what they learned in medical school. Equally, there are some excellent neurologists working within the NHS who have chosen to specialise in epilepsy and are up to speed on the latest developments in treatments. Some family GPs also take a special interest in epilepsy, often because they are managing many patients at their surgery who have it. Who you end up seeing initially will largely depend in the first instance on your GP and who they refer you to for diagnosis and/or care. Depending on the complexity of your epilepsy, you may be referred to one of the very specialised epilepsy clinics (tertiary services or centres of excellence) scattered around the UK that offer extensive diagnostic services and specialist surgeons.

Second opinions

Sometimes consultants can be dismissive of your symptoms and don't provide an accurate diagnosis. Or they may not take your concerns about any prescribed treatment, such as drug side effects, seriously. If you are not happy for any reason, you have the right to ask for a second opinion (although this is not an automatic entitlement). If you want a second opinion, go back to your GP to ask for a new referral. You may find you need to argue your case strongly if there is any reluctance. If so, be prepared to put your emotions to one side and set out the facts as plainly as possible.

Follow-up appointments

Once your diagnosis has been confirmed, you will be given follow-up appointments so the consultant can check up on you at regular intervals. Initially these appointments can be every three or six months, eventually becoming yearly. It is vital that you attend your follow-up appointments – you risk being bumped off the consultant's list if you miss one. If this happens you will need to see your GP and start the referral process again and you may have a very long wait. If you can't attend for any reason, make sure you call to let the clinic know and get a new appointment.

If you respond well to medication and your epilepsy becomes very stable, your consultant may decide you don't need to attend the clinic again. This decision should only be made with your full agreement and you should be offered fast-track access to the consultant if your seizures resume or change. You may need to go through your GP to regain access to the consultant, but your place on their patient list should only ever be on hold and not terminated in such a situation. Your GP should also call you in for an annual review of your care plan.

Epilepsy nurses

At some NHS neurology clinics, where the neurologist specialises in epilepsy, there may also be an epilepsy nurse attached to the service provided. Sometimes known as Sapphire Nurses, they are funded not by the NHS but by Epilepsy Action (one of the main epilepsy charities in the UK).

The role of the epilepsy nurse is to provide support, advice and counselling to anyone with epilepsy and members of their family. The epilepsy nurse will often help to run the epilepsy clinic on the days it is held. Once you have seen your consultant, you can have a chat with the nurse to discuss any aspects of your treatment or care. The nurse may also offer a telephone helpline service if you want to talk anything over in between appointments.

If you don't have access to an epilepsy nurse, the main epilepsy charities provide telephone helpline services if you need to talk about anything or have any questions.

Drugs

Medication is usually the first treatment offered once you have been diagnosed. Depending on the type of epilepsy you have, you will most likely be prescribed one or more anti-epileptic drugs (AEDs) to control your seizures. There is a wide range of AEDs on offer, some of which have been available for decades and some of which are relatively new. You will probably be prescribed tablets but most AEDs are also available in other forms such as a syrup or soluble tablet.

Taking only one AED (monotherapy) is the preferred option for controlling seizures, but sometimes it may be necessary to add in one or more other AEDs to improve control. Your doctor might call this polytherapy, combination therapy, adjunctive therapy or add-on treatment (see glossary).

It can take some time to achieve results with AEDs as you and your consultant may need to experiment with the dosage until any side effects are minimised and you are enjoying a good level of control over your seizures. You might need to try several different AEDs until you find one that is right for you. Around 70% of people achieve full or good control over their seizures on AEDs, so be patient and be prepared to persevere.

It is vital that you take your medication as prescribed, which can be between one and four times a day. Create a routine and stick to it. If you miss a dose, you could put yourself at risk of having a seizure. Also you should never take a double dose to catch up. If you have trouble remembering when to take your medication, you can buy pill containers from the chemist to help you to organise your tablets. If you have an alarm facility on your watch or mobile phone, set this to bleep at the required times to prompt you.

Stomach bugs that cause vomiting or diarrhoea will inevitably interfere with your medication routine. When you and your doctor are preparing your care plan, ask for advice on what to do if you get sick and 'lose' doses as a result.

Weaning

When you first start taking an AED you will probably start on a partial dose and then be asked to increase it gradually over the next few weeks. Being weaned onto your medication helps to minimise any side effects.

Remember to keep a careful note of any side effects – most will disappear once your body has adjusted to being on the full dose, but if not it will help your doctor if you can give a good description of any problems.

If your AED turns out to be unsuitable and you need to try a different one, you will need to wean yourself off the old one and wean onto the new one at the same time. Likewise, if your consultant decides to add in a second drug to improve your seizure control, the new drug will be increased slowly. Your consultant should give you precise instructions for either situation. If you stop medication completely (see page 40), you need to reduce the dose gradually – stopping abruptly can itself trigger a seizure.

Side effects

Almost everyone taking AEDs will experience some side effects. These will most likely be temporary and disappear as your body adjusts to being on the drug, or they may be something you have to learn to live with. All AEDs will have an information leaflet in the box they come in – make sure you read it and know what to expect as typical side effects for your particular prescription. The list may be daunting but remember that you are very unlikely to experience more than a couple of them and they will probably only be mild at that.

Common side effects for many AEDs include:

- Weight gain.
- Mood swings.
- Drowsiness.
- Sore gums.
- Blurred vision.
- Dizziness.
- Memory problems.
- Poor concentration.
- Skin problems such as acne.

You may also experience an allergic reaction to your AED. This usually manifests itself as a skin rash within a matter of days and you should seek urgent advice if this happens. Call your GP or the epilepsy nurse if you have access to one and ask for an emergency appointment with your consultant. Do not stop taking the drug until your doctor has advised you to do so.

Yellow Card Scheme

The Yellow Card Scheme (see help list for contact details) is a way of reporting side effects to the government-run Medicines and Healthcare products Regulatory Agency (MHRA), which is responsible for ensuring the safety of all medications licensed for use in the UK. Reporting side effects helps the MHRA keep tabs on potential emerging problems for a particular medicine. You can find Yellow Card forms at your GP surgery, chemists and hospitals or NHS drop-in centres. You can also fill in the form online on the Yellow Card website or call its hotline.

Continuity of supply

To keep costs down, the NHS encourages doctors to prescribe generic medicines rather than brands. When a new drug is licensed for use, the manufacturer is allowed to provide it exclusively for a certain number of years. At the end of the period, other pharmaceutical companies are allowed to produce generic versions of the drug. The active ingredient (the one that actually helps control your seizures) will always be exactly the same, but the other ingredients that help make up the tablet can vary slightly. It is these variations that cause some people to suddenly experience more side effects or see their seizures return.

NICE guidelines advise that people with epilepsy are entitled to continuity of supply. Your prescription will usually give the generic name of the drug (e.g. levetiracetam), but if your prescription has always been for the branded drug (e.g. Keppra) then you are allowed to continue having this in order to reduce the possibility of any medical problems. This may mean you need to talk to your doctor to ask them to put the brand name on your prescription.

Blood tests

Most AEDs are eliminated from the body through the liver, so your doctor may ask you to have a yearly blood test to check your liver function. Some AEDs are eliminated through the kidneys, so you might have to have a blood test for kidney function too. If you are experiencing severe side effects, you may need to have these tests repeated more frequently.

Blood tests may also be requested to check:

- Whether you are taking the prescribed dose.
- If any side effects are related to the level of your dose.
- Any interaction between your AED and any other medication you have been prescribed.
- If you are pregnant.
- If there is a possibility you have osteoporosis (loss of bone density) which can be aggravated by certain AEDs, particularly if there is a family history of this.

Blood tests will also be requested if you are a candidate for epilepsy surgery. If you have been prescribed phenytoin you will be sent for a regular blood test – this is necessary to ensure you are on the right dosage level. Unfortunately, this is the only way it can be done (the level of phenytoin must be monitored as too high a dose can affect your blood cell count and absorption of certain vitamins or cause phenytoin toxicity).

Alcohol

Alcohol can interfere with the effectiveness of some AEDs or worsen any side effects. You may also find that the combination of AEDs and alcohol means you get drunk very quickly. You will need to weigh up your individual risk if you choose to drink alcohol. For more information on alcohol, see chapter 4.

AEDs for Adults*

The following chart lists all the main AEDs licensed for use in the UK for adults with epilepsy and their common side effects. Other known side effects should be listed on the information leaflet that comes with the AED. More detailed information on all these drugs is available from the main epilepsy charities.

* See chapter 7 for a table of AEDs for children.

Quality of life issues

If you are taking AEDs, many side effects are short-lived as you adjust to being on daily medication while others will persist long-term. Your doctor will always have your overall wellbeing in mind when prescribing, the aim being for you to become completely seizure-free. This may mean a change in prescription if one drug is not really working or increasing the dosage to a higher level. Both these changes could result in increased side effects that you may feel reduce your quality of life. Many AEDs, for example, can have side effects such as persistent tiredness or sleepiness, or loss of concentration.

Only you can weigh such issues in the balance and decide if the side effects are worth the goal of becoming seizure-free, bearing in mind the risks of having seizures. Some people opt to stay on a lower dosage of their AED, with fewer side effects, knowing they could still have one or two seizures a year. Others choose to live with the side effects because it means fewer or no seizures and could possibly have other benefits such as being able to reapply for a driving licence. Your quality of life should always be discussed with your neurologist and major decisions about your level of medication should be achieved jointly.

Generic name	Brand name	Types of seizures	Common side effects
acetazolamide, acetazolomide modified release	Diamox, Diamox SR	Add-on for tonic-clonic and partial seizures. Catamenial epilepsy. Sometimes prescribed for atypical absences, tonic and atonic seizures.	Loss of appetite, drowsiness, depression, pins and needles, joint pain, increased urination, thirst, headaches, dizziness, fatigue, irritability.
Carbamazepine, Carbamazepine modified release	Tegretol, Carbagen SR, Tegretol Retard	Partial and secondary generalised tonic-clonic seizures, primary generalised seizures.	Skin rash, if allergic. Double vision, unsteadiness and nausea if the starting dose is too high.
clobazam	Frisium	Add-on for all seizure types.	Drowsiness.
clonazepam	Rivotril	All seizure types.	Drowsiness.
ethosuximide	Emeside Zarontin	Absence seizures.	Nausea, drowsiness and weight loss (anorexia) if the starting dose is too high.
gabapentin	Neurontin	Monotherapy or add-on for partial seizures with or without secondary generalisation.	Drowsiness, dizziness, headaches.
lacosamide	Vimpat	Add-on for partial-onset seizures with or without secondary generalisation.	Dizziness, headache, nausea, double vision.
lamotrigine	Lamictal	Monotherapy and add-on for partial seizures, primary and secondary generalised tonic-clonic seizures, seizures in Lennox-Gastaut syndrome.	Skin rash, if allergic. Drowsiness, double vision, dizziness, headaches, insomnia, tremors, flu-like symptoms.

levetiracetam	*Keppra*	*Monotherapy and add-on for partial seizures with or without secondary generalisation. Add-on for myoclonic seizures and generalised tonic-clonic seizures.*	*Dizziness, drowsiness, irritability, behavioural problems, insomnia, unsteadiness, tremors, headaches, weight loss (anorexia). Nausea may be experienced at a high dosage or when doses are increased, but this is usually temporary.*
oxcarbazepine	*Trileptal*	*Monotherapy and add-on for partial seizures with or without secondary generalised tonic-clonic seizures.*	*Skin rash, if allergic. Double vision, unsteadiness, headaches, nausea, confusion and vomiting.*
phenobarbital (phenobarbitone)		*All types of epilepsy except absences.*	*Drowsiness, on starting. Persistent lethargy, sedation and slow mental performance.*
phenytoin	*Epanutin*	*All types of epilepsy except absences.*	*Skin rash, if allergic. Drowsiness, unsteadiness, slurring if the dose is too high. Prolonged use can cause coarsening of facial features, overgrowth of gums, excess hair growth, acne and anaemia.*
pregabalin	*Lyrica*	*Add-on for partial seizures with or without secondary generalisation.*	*Dizziness, fatigue, mood swings, loss of concentration, change in appetite, weight gain, blurred/double vision, oedema, drowsiness, speech disorder, memory impairment, confusion and pins and needles.*
primidone	*Mysoline*	*All types of epilepsy except absences.*	*Nausea, unsteadiness, dizziness and drowsiness (on starting). Persistent sedation and slow mental performance.*
rufinamide	*Inovelon*	*Add-on for seizures in Lennox-Gastaut syndrome.*	*Skin rash, if allergic. Dizziness, headaches, nausea, vomiting, drowsiness, fatigue.*

sodium valproate, sodium valproate modified release	Epilim, Orlept, Epilim Chrono, Episenta	All types of epilepsy.	Short-term hair loss (reversible) on starting. Drowsiness, tremors, weight gain, increased incidence of polycystic ovary syndrome and erratic periods. Increased risk of foetal damage if taken in pregnancy.
tiagabine	Gabitril	Add-on for partial seizures with or without secondary generalisation.	Dizziness, fatigue, nervousness, tremors, loss of concentration, depression, agitation.
topiramate	Topamax	Monotherapy and add-on for generalised tonic-clonic seizures or partial seizures with or without secondary generalisation. Add-on for seizures in Lennox-Gastaut syndrome.	Headaches, drowsiness, dizziness, pins and needles, weight loss, kidney stones. Possible temporary speech disorder, impaired memory and concentration on increasing the dose.
valproic acid	Convulex	All types of epilepsy.	Nausea, vomiting and weight loss (anorexia) on starting. Increased appetite, weight gain, gastralgia, gastric spasms, diarrhoea, constipation.
vigabatrin	Sabril	Add-on for partial seizures with or without secondary generalisation not well controlled by other AEDs. Must be initiated and supervised by a specialist. Monotherapy for management of infantile spasms (West's syndrome).	Drowsiness, behaviour, mood swings, psychosis, visual field defects. Visual field tests should be done every six months.
zonisamide	Zonegran	Add-on for refractory partial seizures with or without secondary generalisation.	Skin rash, if allergic. Drowsiness, dizziness, weight loss, kidney stones, confusion, cognitive slowing, agitation, irritability, depression, speech disorders.

Coming off AEDs

Under certain circumstances you may be able to stop taking medication. Your neurologist is most likely to consider this if you have responded so well to an AED, particularly if you have only tried one, that you have remained seizure-free over a period of two to five years. Some people have found that they continue to remain seizure-free after they have stopped taking AEDs. Others find they stay seizure-free for a while but then the seizures return. Again, such a decision needs to be weighed carefully and agreed jointly with your neurologist.

If you decide to go ahead and try living without taking medication, make sure you can regain quick access to your neurologist should your seizures ever return as you will probably need to resume taking AEDs. Never stop taking your AEDs abruptly as this can trigger a seizure – your neurologist should draw up a timetable for you to wean yourself off gradually and you should be offered a follow-up appointment once you have stopped the medication completely.

Brain surgery

Not everyone with epilepsy responds well to medication. If you have tried at least three different AEDs and your seizures remain severe and frequent, your neurologist may suggest brain surgery as an option. However, this is only possible if it's known exactly where in the brain your seizures start. Surgery is generally successful for around 70% of suitable patients.

The route to surgery

If you are a potential candidate for surgery, you will need to have a lot of tests to see if having an operation will help you. You will probably have an EEG test which may involve video telemetry (filming you during the EEG test) plus several brain scans – either MRI or CT – to pinpoint any physical focus of your seizures, such as a tumour, damage from a head injury or scarring of the brain tissue. If the physical cause is evident, further tests will be ordered. These are likely to include physical and psychological tests that will help determine whether surgery might damage any brain functions like speech or memory. How you react to stress will also be investigated as having brain surgery can be very stressful. All these tests can take up to a year or more to complete. Around 50% of people who start pre-surgical testing discover that surgery is not, in fact, an option after all.

Your neurologist will want to be certain that:

- The part of your brain that is the focus of your seizures can be easily reached.
- The specific area can be removed safely.
- You will not lose any important functions such as memory, speech, vision, hearing or motor (movement).
- There is a very high possibility of stopping your seizures or heavily reducing them.

If these criteria can be fulfilled, the test results are good and you have no other medical conditions that rule out brain surgery, then you and your neurologist can discuss whether to go ahead or not.

Making your mind up

You should be given plenty of time to discuss all the risks and benefits, and have any questions answered with your neurologist and also your surgeon if you pass the tests. You have the choice to stop the process at any time. No one will put pressure on you to go ahead as having brain surgery is a huge decision to face. Pre-surgical counselling is offered to help you weigh up everything and make the final decision.

The operation

Your operation is most likely to involve either removing the area of the brain that is causing your seizures, such as a tumour or patch of scarring, or separating the relevant area from the rest of the brain to stop the seizures spreading. The brain has no nerve endings at all, so you could actually be woken up for part of the operation when the surgeon is working on the brain tissue – your conversation and other responses can help the surgeon ensure no important brain functions are being affected.

Recovering

After surgery you may still have seizures for a few days – these will not be epileptic seizures but just the brain readjusting itself following the operation. You may remain in hospital for up to six weeks, depending on how quickly you recover. You will still need to take your AEDs for a while – your neurologist will advise you when and how to start reducing your medication with a view to complete withdrawal from it. You can also expect to have regular reviews with your medical team for up to two years afterwards to track your physical recovery and also your emotional wellbeing – adjusting to a life without seizures can be quite difficult psychologically for some people when it has been life-defining for so long.

Vagus nerve stimulation

Vagus nerve stimulation (VNS) is another surgical option if your epilepsy proves hard to control. Unlike brain surgery, it is not likely to stop your seizures completely but, if successful, it should reduce their frequency and severity.

The vagus nerve communicates essential information between the vital organs (heart, liver, kidneys, etc) and the brain. Stimulating the vagus nerve can reduce blood pressure, heart rate and the frequency of epileptic seizures.

How it works

Under surgery, the left vagus nerve in the neck has three small electrode coils wrapped around it. These are connected to a tiny pulse generator inserted under the skin at the collar bone. The generator is then programmed to stimulate the vagus nerve with electrical pulses, usually for 30 seconds every five minutes on a continuous basis. You also wear or carry a special magnet – if you feel a seizure coming on, the magnet can kick-start extra stimulation to lessen its effects on you.

The surgical process

The operation itself takes a couple of hours and you'll be given a general anaesthetic. The surgeon will make two small incisions – one in the neck for the coils and one on the collar bone to insert the generator. Around a month later, once the incisions have healed, your neurologist will program the generator using a hand-held computer attached to a special wand which is passed over the stimulator to transmit the program.

After surgery

You will need to keep taking your AEDs for some time after having a VNS device inserted. It can take up to two years to see any improvement in the frequency or severity of your seizures. If you do experience an improvement your neurologist should discuss reducing your medication, but you may find you can't stop taking it completely. Your generator can be reprogrammed as needed at follow-up appointments. Its battery lasts for up to 10 years, so you will need further surgery at that point to replace it.

VNS does have some side effects, notably some hoarseness, a tickly throat, coughing, difficulty swallowing and feeling short of breath. Some of these may lessen over time. Using the magnet, it's possible to disable the generator briefly while you eat if swallowing continues to be a problem.

Success rates

Most people opting for VNS find they see at least some improvement in their quality of life. For some people, VNS brings no change – it's possible to have the generator switched off or even removed after two years if this is the case. However, it is not possible to remove the coils around the vagus nerve.

Gamma knife surgery

This is a very new form of surgery that is also called stereotactic radio surgery. It uses gamma radiation to destroy very specific areas of the brain (such as scarring or a benign cyst) that are the focus of your epilepsy. Gamma rays penetrate body tissue, like x-rays, and are therefore good for destroying damaged or dead tissue, like cancerous tumours. No actual surgery is required – your skull will not be opened up.

To date, gamma knife surgery has mostly been used to treat patients who do not have epilepsy but have tumours or other major brain problems. Only a handful of specialist centres in the UK offer gamma knife surgery at present and only a tiny number of people with epilepsy have had it. It's only likely to be offered to you if there are strong reasons for not having conventional brain surgery and it could take up to three years before you see any improvement in your seizures. No figures are available yet for success rates.

Alternative treatments

Medication is the frontline treatment for epilepsy, but it is also possible to manage your seizures using complementary medicine techniques. Many people use these alongside their AEDs, but some choose to use alternative medicine alone. This approach tends to work best if your seizures are triggered by stress as many complementary therapies use a holistic approach to treat the whole person rather than treating only the symptoms, and stress reduction and relaxation forms a part of that.

If you are considering trying to manage your seizures without medication, be sure to discuss this with your neurologist and make any changes with their full support. Before embarking on any such treatments, do thorough research and choose only qualified, reputable practitioners who belong to a professional body that applies standards and monitors its members.

Which therapy?

Complementary therapies can be broadly divided into two camps – those that teach you techniques for relaxing and eliminating stress and those that aim to heal ailments. Whatever you decide to try, and regardless of whether you approach a practitioner about any health issues unrelated to your epilepsy, you need to be honest about having epilepsy and how it affects you.

Known problems

Some products used in complementary medicine can make seizures worse. Certain essential oils used in aromatherapy are known to stimulate the brain and could trigger seizure activity. These include sage, rosemary, sweet fennel and hyssop. Herbal medicine, including Chinese medicine and ayurveda, can also be a problem as some herbs may aggravate your seizures. Be aware too that some nutritional supplements can interfere with your medication and seizure threshold. These include evening primrose oil, starflower oil and St John's wort.

Summing Up

You are most likely to be prescribed one or more anti-epileptic drugs (AEDs) if you have epilepsy. It can take time and perseverance to find the right dose of the right drug but 70% of people do achieve full or near-total control of their seizures using medication. If your seizures do not respond well to medication, you may want to explore the options of surgery or vagus nerve stimulation. Some complementary therapies may help you to reduce stress while others may worsen your seizures.

Managing Your Epilepsy

Learning how to adapt to life with epilepsy can help you to keep your seizures as under control as possible while living life to the full. A large part of managing your epilepsy will centre on minimising risks to yourself. There's no need to wrap yourself in cotton wool – your life would become boring very quickly – but being aware of risks in your day-to-day life as well as for new activities will help you make informed decisions about what you want to do.

Telling people

Deciding how much to tell other people is something you may have to consider repeatedly. It's a good idea to be as open as you can with those closest to you, for example family members or your partner. They will almost certainly want to know if or how they can help you in any way and what to do if you have a seizure in front of them.

Seizure diaries

Keeping a seizure diary can play an important role in managing your epilepsy. You should record as much information as possible about each seizure – the date and time it happened, what type of seizure you had, any possible triggers and any other relevant information such as your mood (were you feeling very stressed or overexcited?), whether you had any illness at the time, changes to your medication (including if you missed a dose), any side effects and any other medication you may be taking. Any information you can remember about the seizure itself, or descriptions if someone else saw it, should also be noted. If you are a woman it can be helpful to record your menstrual cycle as some women find this affects their seizures.

Over a period of time, the diary will show up any obvious patterns for the frequency or severity of your seizures, as well as any possible triggers. This knowledge can help you to avoid any known triggers in the future. Take your seizure diary with you whenever you see your doctor for a review of your treatment as it can help them decide whether you need to make changes to your treatment. Even if your seizures are very infrequent, keeping a diary will ensure you don't lose track of when your last seizure was – this is also information your doctor may want to know.

The main epilepsy charities provide blank seizure diaries that you can download from their websites or buy online. You could also just keep a diary on your computer or in a special notebook.

The example opposite contains actual extracts from the author's own seizure diary.

Reducing stress

Stress does not cause epilepsy but is one of the main triggers for seizures. Studies have proven that stress can cause physiological changes in the brain, increasing your risk of having seizures. Reducing stress as much as possible can therefore be crucial for gaining control over your seizures. It is also the most important self-help treatment, so taking stress reduction seriously and building it in your lifestyle can make a real difference to your quality of life.

Stress is only bad for us when it affects our health. What gives you a racing heart or sweaty palms may not bother the next person at all. Some people thrive under pressure while others crumble. You could have a stressful job full of long hours and tight deadlines and find it doesn't affect your seizures at all, yet others may find their seizures worsen when faced with such pressures. Knowing what makes you feel stressed and how to deal with it can make a big difference to the frequency or severity of your seizures.

Research has also shown that you are more likely to have seizures if you are bored or fed up. Keeping yourself busy and developing hobbies you enjoy will help you relax and possibly keep seizures at bay.

3 October 07 – 10.30am

Tonic-clonic

No warning as usual. Came to on the floor of my office, was very confused as I couldn't understand why the light was on late at night. Slept on the floor for an hour, then woke up and went to bed properly. Woke up with post-ictal headache, threw up.

16 Nov 07 – 10.30am

Tonic-clonic

No warning. Woke up in bed with post-ictal headache. No recollection of anything before that, but think I may have been in the living room.

29 Jan 08 – 11.30am

Simple partial

Mind started racing again with weird thoughts, can't remember any of them. Lasted maybe 10-15 seconds. Felt drained and wanted to throw up but couldn't. Partner helped me to bed, was shivering with cold. Dozed for maybe an hour, had post-ictal headache.

12 June 08 – 10.00am

Tonic-clonic

In the bedroom. Came to on the carpet, where I threw up, mostly saliva. Spent well over 20 mins on the floor drifting in and out of consciousness, then managed to drag myself into bed. Slept until noon. Woke up with very weak limbs, post-ictal headache, painful jaw and carpet burns on face.

8 Aug 08 – 9.35am

Simple partial

Chatting to friend in the hall. Suddenly started feeling weird – could articulate in my head what I wanted to say but couldn't speak. Managed half a sentence: 'think it's epi…'. Couldn't manage any more speech but was perfectly aware of my surroundings and able to understand everything friend was saying. Lasted about two minutes (both our estimate). Speech started to return over next 10 mins but I felt nauseous for two hours after.

25 Jan 09 – around 8.40am

Simple partial

Witnessed by partner. Felt disoriented, tried to converse but couldn't think of words, then felt 'dizzy' and laid on the floor. Lasted about a minute. Felt nauseous afterwards for several hours, with post-ictal headache.

Sleep

Getting enough sleep every night is essential for wellbeing. Most people, whether they have epilepsy or not, need around seven hours per night. Quality of sleep is important too – you should be able to drop off quickly and easily, sleep soundly through the night and wake feeling refreshed. If you have trouble falling asleep and find yourself lying awake fretting about things, or wake frequently during the night, you should consult your GP for help. Tiredness is a major trigger for seizures, yet there are lots of tried and tested remedies for improving your sleep quality (see below). Your GP may be reluctant to prescribe sleeping tablets because of the risk of them interfering with your AEDs, but they can refer you to a specialist for further help if needed.

Tips for developing good sleep habits:

- Stick to a bedtime routine and try to go to bed at the same time each night. Waking at the same time each morning should be part of this.
- Your bedroom should be comfortable and a place only for sleeping. Get rid of any TVs, radios or computer games. Make sure the room is not too hot or too cold and is well ventilated. Don't smoke in the bedroom.
- Before bedtime, try to relax by listening to some gentle music or doing a little yoga. You may find reading for 30 minutes before lights out helps you to settle.
- Make sure you are tired at bedtime. Take some daily exercise (particularly good if you have a non-physical job) or go for a walk in the early evening.
- Avoid stimulants such as coffee, tea, cocoa and alcohol late at night. A warm milky drink can help you feel sleepy, as can some herbal tea blends.
- A light snack before bedtime can encourage sleepiness. Avoid a heavy meal as this can keep you awake while you digest it.

Anxiety

Worrying about things is a major source of stress. If you have problems at work or are concerned about money or your relationship, it may be a good idea to talk to someone appropriate who can help you, such as a debt adviser, your supervisor or a counsellor.

Epilepsy itself can also cause stress. Accepting that you have a life-changing condition can be hard, but stressing about it could make it harder to get under control. It's not unusual to fear having a seizure in public and to worry what other people might think. Unfortunately, this can become a vicious circle – being frightened of having a seizure can trigger one, which in turn aggravates your fear of having another one.

Studies have indicated that some people with certain types of epilepsy are more prone to anxiety and depression. If you feel depressed, talk to your GP and discuss treatments – you may need medication.

Alcohol and recreational drugs

Both alcohol and recreational drugs have a physical impact on the normal functioning of the brain. Both should be approached with caution.

Alcohol

Many people with epilepsy are able to enjoy small amounts of alcohol with no adverse side effects. Others find that even a tiny sip can trigger a seizure. Only you can decide whether to drink or not, depending on how you react to alcohol. Usually one unit (half a pint of beer or a small glass of wine) or two is perfectly safe. You may also discover that your risk of having a seizure comes not from having a drink itself but from the after-effects. Alcohol causes dehydration and if you don't drink plenty of water between alcoholic drinks and then also at bedtime, you will have a hangover on waking which could trigger a seizure. Alcohol also disrupts sleep patterns, so this can be a problem if your seizures are triggered by tiredness.

Alcohol can reduce the effectiveness of almost all anti-epilepsy medications or cause unpleasant but otherwise harmless side effects like hot flushes. Conversely, your AED may also increase the effect of alcohol on you, making you drunk very quickly. Whichever AED you take, check the information leaflet in the box to see what the recommendations are for alcohol consumption.

Bear in mind that some of the newer AEDs have not been available long enough for long-term studies to have been conducted on the effects of alcohol mixed with these medications, so the information leaflet may advise against drinking as a precaution. Again, only you can make a decision not to drink, or to drink and find your safe level.

Drugs

Taking recreational drugs is a very personal decision – you probably already know it is illegal to take drugs and are aware of what some of the physical risks include. Cocaine, amphetamines and ecstasy are all known to increase your chance of having a seizure if you take them. All three are classified as Class A or Class B (the most serious) and are stimulants, meaning you will have trouble sleeping while still high (lack of sleep being itself a trigger for seizures). Studies have shown that long-term use of ecstasy can even trigger epilepsy in someone who has not had it before. The risks that come with drug-taking are therefore very high.

The medical establishment is divided on the use of cannabis. There is no doubt that the 'skunk' (a type of grass) sold in the UK today is far stronger than that available 20 years ago and studies show that long-term use of higher strength cannabis can cause seizures. However, cannabis is also known to have medicinal properties, one of which is as an anti-convulsant.

There is a lot of anecdotal evidence that some people with epilepsy have found cannabis useful in helping control seizures, either in combination with AEDs or on its own. Some people have reported coming off their medication completely and maintaining a seizure-free state through use of cannabis alone. A very limited number of medical studies have been conducted that seem to support this anecdotal evidence. The British Medical Association has stated that it may be useful as an 'adjunctive therapy' for people whose seizures are not completely controlled with conventional AEDs. Cannabis was re-upgraded as an illegal Class B drug in January 2009.

Staying safe in the home and outside

Seizures inevitably increase the risk of injuring yourself, particularly if you have tonic-clonic seizures with no prior warning as this means you have no opportunity to put yourself in a safe place before the seizure starts. It's impossible to eliminate all risks but you can do much to reduce them by considering what could be dangerous and finding practical solutions.

A few tips

Think about the furnishings in your home – you could replace items such as glass-topped tables or furniture that has sharp corners (you can buy protective corner pads). Carpets and rugs provide cushioning if you fall, while non-slip tiles can be laid in kitchens and bathrooms. Fit guards to fireplaces and radiators and lag any exposed hot-water pipes to reduce the risk of burns.

In the kitchen, microwaving is the safest way to cook as the outside does not become hot and it will switch itself off at the end of the cooking time. Frying carries the highest risk. Use the back of the hob and turn panhandles away from where they could be knocked. You can fit cooker guards that stop you falling against the rings or pans.

In the bathroom, showering is safer than bathing as there is less risk of drowning. If you must have a bath, keep the water shallow, have someone in the house and don't lock the door. A baby monitor can alert them to any problems while affording you privacy. Make sure the door opens outwards in case you fall against it.

Gardening and DIY also carry risks, particularly if you need to use ladders or power tools. Again, it is sensible to have company with you.

Living alone

If you live alone you need to give extra consideration to any risks you face and how you might deal with them, such as checking in by phone several times a day with a relative or friend. Make sure someone you trust who lives close by has a spare key to your house. Your local social services can do a safety assessment of your home and even supply you with some safety aids or alarms.

Safety aids

There are many safety gadgets on the market ranging from bed or personal alarms and anti-suffocation pillows to furniture padding and kitchen aids such as cooker guards. What you need will depend on your risk level. A list of suppliers can be found in the help list at the back of this book.

Identity jewellery

When outside the home, it's a good idea to carry some form of medical ID in case you have a seizure. If you are injured, the paramedics will need to identify you quickly and know what medication you are on as well as being able to contact your family. The epilepsy charities can provide simple paper ID cards in a plastic wallet that carry information on your seizure types, medication regime and other vital information. If you have a mobile phone, store 'ICE' ('in case of emergency') in your contacts list with a number for a relative or trusted friend. Paramedics are trained to check phones for an ICE contact.

ID jewellery varies widely in price and format. You can buy bracelets or lockets that contain a paper record of your medical issues, but the disadvantage with these is that space to write your information can be very limited. Some necklaces are inscribed with a telephone number for a 24-hour subscription service – a paramedic who calls the number can access your data to treat you safely. These services can be expensive, with an annual fee.

The newest gadgets on the market are USB flash drives that can be inserted into a hospital computer. The interface can be passworded so only you can change your data, while the casing is stamped with the internationally recognised symbol for medical emergency. Some of these flash drives double as dog-tags which are popular as jewellery with younger people. See the help list for a selection of jewellery suppliers.

Radar keys

A Radar key is a special key that gives you access to public disabled toilets. It's worth applying for one – they cost around £3 – as the extra space in a disabled toilet can lessen your chance of injury if a seizure strikes while you are in the toilet. Having your own Radar key can also spare the embarrassment of having to ask for one at a railway station or shop. Contact DIAL for information on how to acquire one (details can be found in the help list).

Sports and leisure activities

Sport can be very beneficial if you have epilepsy as it can help you stay relaxed. Most sporting activities can be enjoyed if your epilepsy is well controlled, you have assessed the risks and taken any advisable precautions. Some activities are best avoided, while a few are barred unless you have been seizure-free for some time. Check with your doctor if you have any questions.

Safe sports

Team sports such as football, netball or hockey are all safe but you should tell the team manager you have epilepsy and make sure they know what to do if you have a seizure. You may want to wear a safety helmet, particularly for sports like rugby or cycling where there is a risk of head injury. Gentler activities such as rambling, yoga, tai chi and dancing are all reasonably safe.

Working out at the gym should be safe. When processing your membership, gyms always ask about a number of particular health conditions, of which epilepsy is one. You will almost certainly be asked for a doctor's note stating you are fit to train – this is to cover their own insurance needs and without your GP's backing they may not allow you to join. When training, stay hydrated and don't over-exert yourself – either of which could trigger a seizure.

Risky activities

- Boxing, particularly if your epilepsy was caused by head injury.
- Climbing – reduced oxygen at altitudes above 3,500 metres can trigger seizures.
- Extreme sports such as abseiling, paragliding and caving – safety regulations are usually set by governing bodies for these sports, so you will need to do proper research into whether you can participate.
- Scuba diving – you cannot participate at all unless you have been seizure-free for five years and off medication (three years if you have nocturnal seizures).
- Flying – learning to fly is also restricted. You need to be seizure-free – how long for depends on the type of licence you want. The Civil Aviation Authority can advise. Their details can be found in the help list.
- Swimming – never swim alone. Use a pool and inform the lifeguard so they can keep an eye on you. Swimming in open water is high-risk even when you are accompanied as it can be harder to bring you safely to shore when there are currents and hidden depths.
- Boating and fishing – never go alone and always wear a life jacket. Kayaking carries extra risks as kayaks do not right themselves if they capsize.

Funfairs

Some rides at theme parks or funfairs may carry a seizure risk for you, particularly if you have photo-sensitive epilepsy and the ride uses flashing lights. Extreme rollercoasters may be a problem if your seizures are triggered by stress. Otherwise, as long as the rides are fitted with the legally required safety equipment, there's no reason why you can't have a good time enjoying the thrills and spills.

Diet

Eating a healthy and well-balanced diet is important when you have epilepsy. Your brain needs the full complement of vitamins, minerals and other nutrients to function properly, so aim for a good mix of proteins, carbohydrates, fats, fruit and vegetables. It's a good idea to eat regularly too. Whether you opt for three big meals a day or five or six much smaller ones, regular intake of food will help to keep your blood sugar levels stable, lessening the chance of a seizure. For the same reason, eating a little junk food once in a while will do no harm, but a diet heavy in fats, sugar and salt carries extra risks. Apart from weight problems, with the associated risks of heart disease and high cholesterol, a junk diet means yo-yoing blood sugar levels and a lack of good nutrition for your brain.

Dieting

If you need to lose weight for health reasons, make sure you follow a sensible eating plan to avoid unstable blood sugar levels. Your GP can refer you to a nutritionist if you need help and support. Be very wary of crash diets or fad diets that promise rapid weight loss as an unbalanced diet could trigger seizures. And never take diet pills without your doctor's approval – they could interfere with your AEDs.

Adapting the ketogenic diet

The ketogenic diet is a strict regimen for children with severe epilepsy and more information on it can be found in chapter 7. Some adults with hard-to-control seizures have found adapting a version of this diet has helped them. The non-medical version of the ketogenic diet is similar to the Atkins diet in that there is a high intake of proteins and fats and a very restricted intake of carbohydrates. There is no official version of an adapted ketogenic diet for adults – embarking on such a step is best done with the support of your GP or neurologist and a nutritionist to ensure you have a good intake of the necessary nutrients.

Seizure dogs

Like guide dogs for the blind, dogs can also be trained to help people with severe epilepsy. Many people with epilepsy have tales about how their pet dog (or even cat) seems to 'just know' when they are going to have a seizure and will start pawing at them or barking. It is not really understood how animals can sense an imminent seizure, but they probably pick up on tiny physiological or behavioural changes, such as someone's smell or their pupils dilating, that are undetectable to humans.

A charity called Support Dogs trains seizure alert dogs specifically to predict the onset of a seizure. They are particularly useful if you have uncontrolled tonic-clonic seizures without auras as you can put yourself in a safe place before your seizure kicks in. Each dog is trained to give you a warning period of at least 20 minutes, which will always be the same length of time for consistency, and to always warn you in the same way, such as barking or jumping up.

As with guide dogs, training is rigorous and best suited to certain breeds, so it is not possible to have your own pet trained. When a dog has reached a certain level of training, they are matched to a prospective owner to complete their training together for seizure recognition. When the dog is fully qualified, it can wear the official yellow 'assistance dog' jacket and has the same legal status as guide dogs and hearing dogs. To find out if you qualify for a seizure alert dog, contact Support Dogs – details can be found in the help list.

Summing Up

Managing your epilepsy involves assessing your own personal level of risk according to how well controlled your seizures are and their type, and taking appropriate practical steps to ensure your safety. Most day-to-day activities should be easily manageable, although you may find you need some aids and gadgets to assist you.

Travel Issues

Driving

You are not allowed to drive in the UK if you have seizures, and the rule applies even if you've only had one seizure and haven't been diagnosed with epilepsy. This is because the risk of causing an accident is very high if you have a seizure while driving. If you have epilepsy, the rule covers all types of seizure including nocturnal ones, regardless of whether you lose consciousness or not. Learner drivers are covered by the same rule.

Losing your driving licence can be a bitter blow. It may mean losing your independence, particularly if you live somewhere not covered by public transport, or even the loss of your livelihood if you drive for a living. These matters can be very hard to come to terms with, although you may regain your licence if your seizures stop. Remember, it is your responsibility to stop driving immediately and to inform the DVLA, the government agency that licenses drivers.

You can get comprehensive information on all the following issues directly from the DVLA. Their contact details can be found in the help list.

Stopping driving

Your doctor should advise you fully, but as soon as you have had a seizure you are legally bound to inform the DVLA. They will then ask you to return your licence to them as it will now be invalid. Continuing to drive is a criminal offence and offenders face stiff penalties – in 2008, the English courts jailed a man for eight years and banned him from driving for 10, after he failed to inform the DVLA that he had nocturnal seizures and subsequently killed a pedestrian when he had a seizure at the wheel. Your insurance will also become invalid.

The DVLA tends to look more favourably on you if you hand your licence back voluntarily rather than them having to contact you. This could make a big difference if you find yourself in a position to reapply for your licence.

Exceptions

You do not need a driving licence if you are driving on private land – the DVLA regulations apply only to the public highways. You can continue to drive the following vehicles as long as you are not on the roads, although some of these may still be covered by health and safety regulations:

- Farm vehicles like tractors.
- Forklift trucks.
- Quad bikes.
- Sit-on lawnmowers.

Reapplying for your licence

The rules for resuming driving vary as follows:

- Group 1: if you had a licence to drive a car, moped or motorbike, you can reapply if you have been seizure-free for 12 months with or without taking AEDs. You will be given a licence for one, two or three years to start with (if you stay seizure-free for seven years, you can apply for a long-term licence). If you have nocturnal seizures only, you can reapply after three years. If you surrendered your licence voluntarily, you can reapply two months before the full year is up (processing the paperwork can take up to two months). You may start driving after 12 months and before you receive the licence, provided that you have checked with the DVLA that your reapplication was received and your doctor agrees that you meet the regulations. If your licence was revoked, you may not start driving again until you have received your new licence.

- Group 2: LGV and PSV drivers (lorries and buses) – you must remain seizure-free without medication for a minimum of 10 years before you can reapply. The DVLA will check with your doctors that you are unlikely to have seizures again.
- Taxi drivers: hackney carriages and minicabs both fall under Group 1 but Local Authorities (LAs) set the regulations for licensing taxi drivers, so you will need to check with your council for any additional requirements on top of DVLA rules.

If your reapplication is refused, the DVLA must explain why. You also have the right to appeal. You must do this in writing within six months at a magistrate's court in England or Wales (Scotland: 21 days at the sheriff's court). You will almost certainly need a letter of support from your GP or neurologist to give weight to your appeal.

Insurance

If you have successfully reapplied for your driving licence, insurance companies are not allowed to discriminate against you by weighting your premium or refusing you a policy just because you have had epileptic seizures. They are, however, allowed to ask for further information about your medical history in order to provide you with a quote. They may also ask for a copy of your licence or confirmation from the DVLA that you are now fit to drive. If you think you have been discriminated against, epilepsy is covered under the Disability Discrimination Act and you can obtain advice from the Equality Commission (details can be found in the help list).

Driving abroad

Driving rules in other countries vary enormously. Even if you successfully reapplied to drive in the UK, you may not be allowed to in other countries. Within the EU, your UK driving licence is valid in all member states. If you plan to drive abroad outside the EU, you will need to check with each country's consulate. Remember that wherever you drive outside the UK, DVLA rules still apply to you – you must inform the DVLA and surrender your licence if you have a seizure abroad.

Public transport

Railcards and bus passes

Help is at hand for getting around without a car, either subsidised or free. Travel passes can be applied for when a disability means you would be refused a driving licence. You normally have to provide written proof with your application that you have epilepsy, such as a copy of your prescription for AEDs, a letter from the DVLA or an award letter stating you are entitled to certain disability benefits. Check the individual requirements for each pass.

Disabled Persons Railcard

The Disabled Persons Railcard costs £18 for one year or £48 for three years (prices correct at time of writing) and gives you a one-third reduction on rail fares (some restrictions may apply on routes and times). The card also entitles one person travelling with you to enjoy the discount too (regulations assume a travelling companion acts as your carer). You can pick up a leaflet from most railway stations or apply through the Railcard website (see help list).

Bus passes

If you live in England, Wales or Scotland, you can apply for a concessionary bus pass from your Local Authority (LA) – this entitles you to free off-peak bus travel on local bus services (and across the whole country). Before 9.30am, a half-fare applies. Londoners can apply for a Freedom Pass that gives free travel on the local trains, tubes and trams. In some other cities, such as Manchester, your local pass can be used for free off-peak travel on local trains and trams. If you live outside London but visit regularly, it's worth getting an Oyster Card for tube travel. You can top it up on a 'pay as you go basis', but if you have a disabled railcard you can have it 'appended' to your Oyster Card and gain a one-third discount on non-bus local transport fares. Concessionary bus passes do not apply to intercity coach travel with companies such as National Express. However, some coach companies do offer disabled discounts, so check with them to see if you are eligible.

Northern Ireland

If you have been refused a driving licence as a result of your epilepsy, you can apply for a Half-Fare SmartPass which entitles you to half-fares on scheduled bus and rail services operating within Northern Ireland. You can get an application form at main bus and rail stations or from the Driving & Vehicle Agency NI.

Other transport help

If your epilepsy is too severe to manage public transport, there are lots of local community schemes like Dial-A-Ride that offer assisted lifts. The Community Transport Association website has a full list, or ask social services for details of local schemes (see help list for details).

Travelling abroad

Travelling outside the UK brings its own set of considerations to ensure your trip remains problem-free, with no or minimal health concerns. Most travel is unlikely to be problematic, but here are some handy tips:

- Make sure you stay rested and hydrated on flights and try not to get too stressed to avoid triggering a seizure.
- There's not much you can do about jetlag except allowing extra time to sleep it off if necessary.
- Cabin crews are trained in first aid procedures, but you might want to warn them if you think a seizure could be a possibility.

Medication

Make sure you have enough medication for your whole trip plus some extra just in case, and carry it in your hand luggage as suitcases can go astray in transit. Keep your tablets in the original packaging – this should minimise problems if you get stopped by customs, but you may also want to bring an explanatory letter from your doctor if there's a possibility of problems importing your AEDs into your destination. Take a spare prescription in case an emergency means you need to acquire more medication.

If your medication is in liquid form, remember that airport security restrictions mean you can only carry liquids in containers of below 100ml. You will need to obtain permission from both the airport and the airline to carry a larger amount onto a plane, as well as supporting documentation from your GP or consultant.

A short hop over the Channel is unlikely to cause major problems for when you take your medication, but as soon as you cross two or more time zones it can be easy to lose track of when it's time for a dose. Carrying two watches, with one still set to UK time, or using the alarm facility on your mobile phone can resolve this issue. The further you travel, the more important it is for you to consider gradually adjusting your medication times so that you don't need to wake yourself in the night to take a tablet.

Most doctors will not write prescriptions to cover more than three months' worth of medication, so if you are planning a lengthy trip, make sure you see your GP or consultant to discuss this – it's possible for them to forward a private prescription to one of the companies that can export medication to you, assuming your destination country has an import licence for your particular AEDs. If you are travelling outside the EU, check in advance that you will be able to obtain your prescription locally – not all AEDs are available in other countries and you may have to reconsider your travel plans.

Vaccinations

Vaccinations are compulsory for certain diseases in many countries and most do not cause any problems if you have epilepsy. Anti-malaria treatments are a problem, however. Chloroquine and Larium are known to cause seizures in some people, while other malarial drugs can interfere with the effectiveness of your AEDs. Anti-malaria drugs that are known to be problem-free are proguanil (Paludrine, Malarone), atovaquone (Malarone), doxycycline (Vibramycin) and pyrimethamine or dapsone (Maloprim). If you can't change your travel plans, seek specialist advice from an NHS vaccination centre.

Insurance

If you are visiting an EU country, plus Iceland, Liechtenstein, Norway and Switzerland, you can access basic free or reduced-cost healthcare (you must have a European Health Insurance Card or EHIC). The scheme is free and is reciprocal with the NHS. You can pick up an application form from a post office or download one from the EHIC website (see help list). Depending on the country and what treatment you have, you may be able to reclaim some costs on your return. While this is very handy and can cover you for minor patch-ups in casualty or GP visits to your hotel if you get sick, it is no substitute for proper travel insurance for healthcare. For example, EHIC will not cover repatriation costs if you become so ill you need to be flown home.

Unfortunately, health insurance premiums are generally higher when you have any kind of long-term health condition. Not all companies distinguish between people with well-controlled epilepsy who are unlikely to need medical attention and people whose seizures are less predictable. Not declaring your epilepsy could render your policy invalid, so you must be honest when filling in the forms. Shop around as policy prices can vary enormously and give as much information as you can about your seizure type, frequency and severity.

Some companies specialise in travel policies for long-term health conditions and these may be better value than buying standard ones. It is also best to avoid buying a policy as part of a package holiday as you may find you are not covered for many things. If you book a package trip, buy your policy separately to get the right deal.

Summing Up

You are not legally allowed to drive in the UK if you have seizures, although you can reapply for a driving licence after being seizure-free for 12 months. Professional drivers face additional restrictions for regaining a licence.

Concessionary passes are available for free or discounted bus or rail travel. If you plan to travel abroad, you need to consider various issues – taking your medication with you, vaccinations, insurance and the stress of the travel itself.

Women and Parenthood

This chapter is mostly aimed at women (including girls) but some information below applies to men too, and there is also a special section on fatherhood.

Hormones and the menstrual cycle

Women are affected in additional ways by epilepsy because of how the hormonal cycle can influence seizures. The two main female sexual hormones – oestrogen and progesterone – regulate periods and pregnancy. Levels of both hormones fluctuate throughout the month, determining the stages of the menstrual cycle. They also have an effect on the brain which can interact with a woman's seizure patterns.

As a result of hormonal activity, some women may develop epilepsy during puberty. Girls who were diagnosed with epilepsy in childhood may see their seizure types and patterns change from adolescence. Changing hormone levels during the menopause can also affect seizures.

About one in three women with epilepsy have seizures that are linked directly to the menstrual cycle. This is known as catamenial epilepsy. If this applies to you, you may have already noticed that you only have seizures during your period, during ovulation or at another predictable point in your cycle. Keeping a seizure diary as well as a menstrual diary will quickly show you if there is a link between the two and can help your doctor decide on the most appropriate treatment. You are likely to be prescribed a combination of AEDs to control this kind of seizure pattern – one to be taken daily and an additional one to be taken at the point in your cycle when you usually have seizures.

Contraception and fertility issues

Anti-epileptic medication can affect contraceptives that rely on hormones to alter your fertility level. This includes all forms of the pill, as well as implants, patches and vaginal rings. Not all AEDs affect hormonal contraceptives, just those that are known as 'enzyme-inducing' – these break down artificial hormones in the body at a faster rate than normal, making your contraceptives less effective. The following AEDs are enzyme-inducing:

- Carbamazepine.
- Oxcarbazepine.
- Phenobarbital.
- Phenytoin.
- Primidone.
- Rufinamide.
- Topiramate.

If you are taking any of these to control your epilepsy and also use the pill or another type of hormonal contraception, your risk of accidental pregnancy increases. You should discuss your medication and contraception needs with your neurologist as you may need to change your AEDs or use other contraceptives. These could include condoms, an IUD (a coil which is inserted into the womb and prevents an embryo from implanting itself and starting a pregnancy), a cap or diaphragm.

Lamotrigine

Lamotrigine (Lamictal) is not an enzyme-inducing AED and it is known not to have long-term effects on fertility. For this reason, it is often prescribed to women of childbearing age for seizure control. However, not all women can take lamotrigine as it is not uncommon to have an allergic reaction to it when starting it. While lamotrigine does not affect the effectiveness of the pill or other hormonal contraceptives, research suggests that the pill may reduce the effect of lamotrigine by lowering its active level in the blood, meaning your chance of having a seizure increases if you are taking this AED as well as the pill.

Lamotrigine also does not combine well with the mini-pill, patches and implants. If you have good seizure control on lamotrigine, you should consider alternative contraceptive methods.

The morning-after pill

You are likely to need emergency contraception (the morning-after pill) if you have had unprotected sex. This can be prescribed by a GP or family planning clinic. Some pharmacists can also prescribe it. If you take an enzyme-inducing AED for your epilepsy (see previous list), you must tell the person who is prescribing for you as you will need to take double the normal dose for it to be effective in preventing a pregnancy.

Planning your family

Having epilepsy does not mean you can't have children, but your family should be planned with the support of your doctors to minimise any potential problems. If you plan to get pregnant, you may want to have counselling beforehand so you can make informed decisions on the options available to you. If you find you have become pregnant unexpectedly, arrange to see your neurologist as soon as possible.

Birth defects

Having epileptic seizures can slightly increase the risk of your child having birth defects. but it's very important to remember that 95% of women with epilepsy who have children have trouble-free pregnancies. You may need to change your AEDs to something more suitable that will not damage the baby in the womb – it can take several months to make the switch successfully.

Sodium valproate (Epilim) is the AED most likely to cause problems with the foetus while carbamazepine (Tegretol) carries a slightly higher risk. Both these AEDs can lead to a higher possibility of neural tube defects (such as spina bifida or cleft lip/palate) while sodium valproate is the drug most associated with foetal anti-convulsant syndrome (FACS) which can cause developmental, behavioural and learning difficulties. Your neurologist should advise you on the kinds of foetal problems associated with each AED.

PCOS

Some women taking AEDs find they develop polycystic ovary syndrome (PCOS) as a side effect of their medication. PCOS can make it hard to conceive but can be treated. It just may take longer to get pregnant. You should be offered a check-up to determine if you have PCOS or not.

Pregnancy

Before becoming pregnant

Once your neurologist has given you the go-ahead to get pregnant, you should stop smoking if you smoke, follow current guidelines for the safe consumption of alcohol and start taking folic acid. All women are advised to take folic acid before and during pregnancy as it helps to prevent neural tube defects in the baby. This is very important if you have epilepsy because of the increased risk of neural tube defects. Your GP should prescribe this for you – if you have applied for a prescription exemption certificate, it won't cost you anything.

AEDs – to take or not?

Prior to becoming pregnant, you may have already changed your AEDs on the advice of your neurologist. If your seizures are uncontrolled, you should be on the lowest possible dose of your medication during the pregnancy so as to minimise any possible adverse effects on your baby. However, once you are pregnant, the changes your body goes through mean you actually need more medication to prevent seizures, so finding the right dose is a very delicate balancing act. Your neurologist should send you for regular blood tests during pregnancy to check your dosage levels are good and monitor any changes in your seizure pattern.

If you have been seizure-free for several years on your medication, you and your neurologist should discuss the possibility of an AED-free pregnancy. The benefit is the reduced possibility of birth defects for your baby. The downside is the risk that your seizures return during your pregnancy and that you or your baby suffer injuries as a result. You should also bear in mind the knock-on effects, such as losing your driving licence again.

Morning sickness

Not all women suffer morning sickness in pregnancy. If you do, consult your neurologist about the possibility of changing the times of the day you usually take your AEDs and what remedies you can safely take to reduce nausea. Morning sickness usually stops after the first trimester (this is the first 12 weeks of your pregnancy) – at this point you'll need to see the neurologist again to discuss adjusting your AEDs.

Tests

During your pregnancy, you are likely to be offered various tests to check how your baby is developing. These tests can detect birth defects such as spina bifida or FACS (see page 82). You should have counselling first to talk through the implications of going ahead or not with any tests, and how you might deal with the outcome if problems are detected during the pregnancy or only discovered at birth.

Vitamin K

Your GP or neurologist may prescribe vitamin K during the last few weeks of your pregnancy. Certain AEDs can reduce the clotting action of the blood, whereas vitamin K improves this. Some babies are born with low levels of vitamin K and have a higher risk of haemorrhages, so taking vitamin K as a supplement should reduce the chance of this happening. Your baby is likely to be injected with a shot of vitamin K within a month of the birth as a booster.

Giving birth

Your midwifery team should be informed of your seizure types, their frequency, your seizure triggers and what AEDs you take. You must bring your medication along to the hospital and take it as normal during labour.

It's very likely you will have a perfectly normal delivery, although there is a 1-2% chance that you may have a tonic-clonic seizure during labour, even if this is not your usual kind. Your midwife should administer drugs to stop the seizure if this happens.

Despite the small chance of a seizure happening during labour, home births are not recommended because in an emergency your midwife may not be able to get you to hospital on time for medical intervention.

Pain relief

If your breathing exercises are not helping and you need pain relief during labour, you may be offered an epidural or gas and air. Many hospitals also offer TENS units which use electrical impulses to ease pain – these are perfectly safe for you and your baby. A TENS (transcutaneous electrical nerve stimulation) unit looks a little like a Slendertone box, with sticky electrode pads that you put on the skin and which transmit the pulses to ease pain. The other main painkiller used in labour is pethidine, however you shouldn't be offered it as this is known to trigger seizures.

After the birth, your neurologist should advise you on gradually adjusting your AEDs if the amount you took before pregnancy was altered during the pregnancy.

Caring for your baby

Breastfeeding

Breastfeeding is safe even when you are taking AEDs. Your baby will have already been exposed to your medication while in the womb and the amount of AEDs in breast milk is very small. Read the leaflet that comes with your AEDs – it should contain comprehensive information about any breastfeeding risks associated with that drug.

While breastfeeding, you may want to consider expressing your milk for night-time feeds – not only is it a way for your partner to be involved with feeding but it will ensure you get a good night's rest. Remember, sufficient sleep is an important way of managing your epilepsy.

Keeping your baby safe

If your seizures are active, you need to consider how you can protect your child. Chapter 4 offers practical advice on sleep, diet and stress reduction to help keep seizures at bay. As a new parent, these matters take on greater importance when coping with the extra stresses of childcare.

Other tips include the following:

- Involve your partner as much as you can in caring for your baby and accept any help offered from family members or friends, particularly if you are tired.
- To reduce the risk of dropping the baby, you can do many things on the floor – changing nappies, feeding or dressing them. If you need to carry your baby, use a padded sling or car seat rather than holding them in your arms.
- Do not bathe your child on your own because of the risk of drowning. If you are alone, give your baby a sponge-down on a mat on the floor instead.
- Make sure whatever buggy you purchase has a brake on it that is activated if the handle is released. Other gadgets you may find helpful include stair gates, baby reins and fireguards.
- Make sure you keep your AEDs, and all other medicines, out of reach from your child.

Your child as your carer

As your child starts to grow up, you can start teaching them what to do if you have a seizure. Children can start learning simple stuff from the age of two or three, like how to dial 999 or that they should stay by your side 'if Mummy falls down'. If you have a medical ID card or special jewellery, you can teach your child to show this to someone if you have a seizure outside the home. By four or five they should be able to find someone and ask for help, and even learn the first aid procedures for seizures.

Menopause

As you enter the menopause, your levels of oestrogen and progesterone will start to fall and your menstrual cycle will start to slow down before stopping completely. You may see changes in your weight which can affect the efficiency of your AEDs and your periods may become erratic (you should monitor this if you have catamenial epilepsy). You could also find that your seizures become frequent as a result of changing hormone levels. Again though, keeping a seizure diary will help track new patterns.

After the menopause, your seizures may return to their previous frequency or even become less frequent. Your neurologist should review your medication, taking into account all of these factors.

Depending on the symptoms of your menopause, you may be prescribed hormone replacement therapy (HRT) which contains synthetic oestrogen. In a very few cases, the oestrogen in HRT may trigger seizures. If your doctor is considering offering you HRT, you should talk through all the possibilities of how this may affect your epilepsy, particularly if your AED is lamotrigine as this is known to interact negatively with HRT. If you go ahead and your seizures change in any way for the worse, see your neurologist.

Many women choose to manage their menopausal symptoms naturally. Some herbal supplements that are freely available over the counter in pharmacies and health stores claim to ease the menopause. As with other herbal remedies, some herbs are known to trigger seizures. If you decide to go down the natural route, make sure you see a qualified herbalist and tell them you have epilepsy.

Osteoporosis (weakening of the bones, leading to breakages) affects many women during and after the menopause as calcium levels drop in the body. If you take an enzyme-inducing AED, you should have a bone density scan to check for signs of osteoporosis as this type of AED is known to reduce bone density.

You should also take supplements of calcium and vitamin D, both of which can help keep your bones strong, and have a blood test every couple of years to check your levels of these. HRT can help protect against osteoporosis but carries its own risk of worsening your seizures.

Fatherhood

The following section is aimed at men who have epilepsy. Their partners may find it helpful too.

Fertility issues

Most men with epilepsy do not have any related fertility problems. However, AEDs can have certain effects on your sex life that may affect your partner's ability to conceive. Side effects can include the loss of your sex drive or the ability to achieve or sustain an erection. If you are experiencing any of these, talk to your GP or neurologist as a change to your medication may make a positive difference.

Certain AEDs are known to affect the quality and amount of sperm you produce. If you are taking carbamazepine, oxcarbazepine, phenobarbital, phenytoin, primidone, sodium valproate or topiramate and your partner is struggling to conceive, you should ask to have a fertility test. If the results are poor, you should be offered any appropriate treatments and advice.

Although women with epilepsy have a slight risk of passing on birth defects, men taking AEDs do not.

Caring for your child

If your seizures are uncontrolled, you may feel nervous about taking care of your child if your partner is not around to help. Many dads, with or without epilepsy, worry about caring for a small baby – this is perfectly natural and parenting is a job you will learn as you go. When you have epilepsy as well, there are extra issues to consider so that you can ensure your child is as safe as possible if you have a seizure.

Read the section on keeping your baby safe for some tips and advice on the practical things you can do to minimise any risks. Your partner may want reassurance that you can manage the childcare safely in her absence – talk over any worries or issues that arise and agree on any necessary compromises.

Summing Up

Women tend to be affected more by epilepsy because of their hormonal cycles from puberty to the menopause. Sometimes the menstrual cycle itself triggers seizures. Epilepsy treatments for women generally take the hormonal effect into account.

If you are hoping to have a family, the pregnancy needs careful advance planning, with the support of your neurologist in order to minimise any risk of birth defects in the baby or problems during the pregnancy or labour.

If you are a mother or father and have epilepsy, you need to consider the safety risks to your child if you have uncontrolled seizures. There are lots of practical steps you can take to do this and there is no reason why epilepsy should prevent you from being a good parent.

Children with Epilepsy

Epilepsy most commonly starts in childhood, although adults can develop it too. Children have the same types of seizures as adults do and many children grow out of it in their teens and are able to stop taking medication. Around 80% of children diagnosed lead reasonably normal lives.

There are certain epilepsy syndromes that are seen only in children. Children with more severe syndromes may face educational problems as a result of their particular health issues or miss classes in order to attend medical appointments. Some children with epilepsy also have other disabilities that can result in learning difficulties or developmental problems.

Is it epilepsy?

When children fall ill they can display epilepsy-like symptoms that aren't actually linked to epilepsy. For example, teething babies or children under the age of five with a viral or bacterial infection may have convulsions that suggest a tonic-clonic seizure. However, febrile convulsions are the more likely cause, especially if coupled with a raised temperature.

Febrile convulsions are non-epileptic seizures that occur when a child's temperature is too high. They rarely cause brain damage or lead to epilepsy and the child will probably outgrow them by the age of four or five. Sometimes children hold their breath when angry or frustrated until they faint. This can be frightening to see, especially if they go blue in the face, but this kind of behaviour is not epilepsy. It shouldn't harm them and the only treatment they are likely to need, if any, is counselling with a suitable therapist if they have experienced trauma.

If your child has any sort of unexpected convulsion or collapses for no obvious reason, seek medical help quickly. Your GP, paramedics or hospital paediatricians should consider epilepsy as a potential diagnosis when other possible conditions have been ruled out.

Spotting symptoms – advice for parents and teachers

Epilepsy is hard to diagnose and symptoms are not always as obvious as convulsions. Partial seizures in particular can display a very wide array of symptoms. Some clues that might suggest epilepsy include the following:

- Your child seems clumsy and drops things, especially if their hands or legs seem to jerk.
- Daydreaming – all children daydream but sometimes what appears to be daydreaming is in fact your child having an absence seizure. If the daydreaming is persistent and your child is also falling behind at school, this could be a clear indicator of absences and you should ask your GP to run tests.
- Blacking out and falling over, either rigidly or limply, could be a sign of tonic or atonic seizures if this happens several or more times.
- Your child complaining of being able to taste or smell things that aren't there, or hearing or seeing things – all these could be indicators of temporal lobe epilepsy.
- Physical tics such as plucking at clothing, smacking the lips or wandering off in a daze and not being able to remember how they got somewhere.

It can be hard not to panic when you see your child behaving strangely but try to keep cool and be a good observer – your doctor will appreciate any descriptions you can give in order to rule epilepsy in or out. Chapter 1 gives in-depth information on symptoms of specific seizure types and how diagnosis is reached.

Childhood epilepsy syndromes

There are many epileptic syndromes and some of them are specific to childhood. These include syndromes such as benign rolandic epilepsy and childhood absence epilepsy, both of which your child has a good possibility of growing out of by puberty or mid-teens. Others, such as Lennox-Gastaut syndrome, can be difficult to both diagnose and treat and your child has a higher likelihood of developmental delay or learning difficulties if they have such syndromes. (See glossary for further details.)

Your paediatrician will inform you if your child has an epilepsy syndrome and you should be given information on how to care for them, as well as treatment options and the long-term outlook. Some syndromes also have their own support organisation where you can talk to other parents coping with the same issues. Your paediatrician or epilepsy nurse may have information on specific syndrome support groups or you can call one of the helplines run by the main epilepsy charities for contact details.

Explaining things to your child

Children understand a surprising amount from an early age and they are often also very accepting of their health problems. You know your child best and you will know when is a good time to start telling them more about their epilepsy. From as early as age two or three, children can start absorbing information and understand why they need to take their medicine. If they ask questions, answer them simply and honestly at a level appropriate for their age and development.

It can be tempting to be very protective of your child but, unless they have very severe disabilities, you should try to encourage them gradually to take responsibility for managing their epilepsy as they grow up. Caring for your child when they have epilepsy can be very stressful but try not to show this to them. Your child will be more keen to take an active role in managing their health if you can present an upbeat outlook. Many of the epilepsy charities can offer useful advice on explaining things and helping your child to take care of him or herself.

Educational issues

The vast majority of children with epilepsy attend school normally and may only need minimal assistance with their schoolwork, like some help catching up if they miss a lesson because they had a seizure. Children with more severe epilepsy may have learning difficulties and require extra support. Educational needs are covered by the Disability Discrimination Act – your child has the right to equal access to schooling.

Working with the school

Some schools have official policies on managing epilepsy, but many do not. Whatever the situation, you should talk to your child's teachers and the school nurse about your child's epilepsy as their understanding of the condition may be sketchy. You may need to explain to school staff that they probably don't need to call for an ambulance every time your child has a seizure, or to send them home, as many children recover quickly and may only need a brief lie-down in the nurse's room. If your child regularly goes into status, the school may need to store emergency medication on the premises. A member of staff should be trained in how to administer it.

In term time your child's teachers will spend more time with your child than you do and are in a good position to spot any changes in your child's wellbeing or notice if they start falling behind in class. If your paediatrician has advised your child to avoid certain activities, inform the school of these. Otherwise, there is no reason your child should not participate fully in all school activities. However, they may need extra supervision in PE or swimming lessons and other classes like science if chemicals are being handled.

Bullying

Children who are different often get picked on in school by other children. The bullying may amount to no more than some name-calling in the playground but it may become worse. If your child is the quiet type, they may have problems asserting themselves and nipping any bullying in the bud. Signs to look out for include reluctance to go to school, truancy, behavioural changes such as moodiness or tearfulness, bedwetting, nervousness, sudden flashes of anger or aggression.

Most schools have a written policy on bullying. Talk to the teachers if you suspect there may be a problem. Your child will need support to stand up for themselves and the school should be able to offer practical solutions such as ensuring your child has friends around them, as well as dealing directly with the bullies. See *Bullying – A Parent's Guide* (Need2Know) for further information.

Learning difficulties

Most children with epilepsy have no problem learning at the same pace as their classmates, even if they miss the occasional lesson because they've had a seizure. However, children who have absence seizures are more likely to fall behind. A child may have tens of absence seizures, or even hundreds, every day, where they are briefly unconscious for up to half a minute and appear to be daydreaming. While they are absent they will be missing out on whatever is happening around them, including hearing information. If the child is undiagnosed, their behaviour may be interpreted as laziness or lack of application. If a diagnosis has been made, the school should provide extra support to help your child stay up to speed in class. Once your child is on medication to control the absences, they will find it much easier to keep up with the other children.

Learning disabilities and special educational needs

Children with more severe epilepsy are more likely to have serious learning problems, especially if they have other disabilities too. Your child could have a poor memory or difficulty concentrating either as a direct result of their epilepsy or because of side effects from their medication.

Most disabled children benefit from being in mainstream education and the school should provide appropriate extra assistance such as remedial classes or a designated classroom assistant to work specifically alongside your child. Your school may have a special educational needs (SEN) adviser who can draw up a framework for helping your child. Otherwise, you should contact the Local Education Authority (LEA) to talk to the SEN officer.

Your child may need to be 'statemented' – this means that your child will be given a statutory assessment and then a written statement will be drawn up of their precise special educational needs. The statement should contain information not just on classroom help but other matters such as regular reviews of your child's progress and setting long-term goals for your child's education so they can still reach their full potential.

The statement may recommend that your child attend a special school. You have the right to choose a school for your child – your decision may be affected by whether your preferred choice has suitable policies in place to support your child. The LEA may not support your first choice, but it must give its reasons in writing and these should normally be related to the fact that the placement would not be appropriate for your child's needs, the needs of other pupils there or that the LEA's resources mean your child can be better helped in another school.

The SEN system is very complex to negotiate and you may need a lot of patience and persistence to ensure your child's schooling needs are met. The LEA should have parent support advisers to help you understand how the SEN framework operates, but you may also choose to get independent support from an organisation such as Advisory Centre for Education (ACE). You can also read *Special Educational Needs – A Parent's Guide* (Need2Know) for further information.

Exams and assessments

Your child may need extra help when it comes to exams. This may include having additional time to prepare in advance if they have missed lessons or extra time while sitting the test if they are slow with reading and writing. Sometimes just knowing a test is imminent can be stressful enough to trigger seizures – some children even fear having a seizure during the exam itself. Examination bodies can make adjustments for children with epilepsy but they will need information from the school, you and your child and possibly your child's doctors too in order to reach appropriate decisions.

Access arrangements are a form of compensation for children who need extra time to sit a test, and up to 25% extra time can be allowed. Your child could have a teaching assistant sit by them to assess their needs during the exam, such as noting if they are having absences or if they need rest breaks. Exam times or locations can also be changed to suit your child's needs if appropriate. It is much easier to get access arrangements if your child already has a SEN statement.

Special consideration is another form of help where children can be awarded up to 5% of their overall marks in the exam. However, special consideration is only given in severe cases, for example where a child has a seizure before an exam. Pupils with epilepsy are usually better off applying for access arrangements. Your child's school and the LEA can advise you of procedures for both these and help you choose which one to ask for.

Medication

Most of the drugs prescribed to control epilepsy in adults are suitable for children under the age of 12. However, children may have slightly different side effects from those experienced by adults. Some child AEDs are only licensed for use in children over a certain age. See the table overleaf for a list of child AEDs (this is a guide only - please see your healthcare team for professional advice).

Child doses of AEDs are much smaller than adult doses and they need to be carefully calculated. Dosages are based on a child's weight in kilos and the prescription will be for so many milligrams per day, per kilo. The total number of daily milligrams will then be divided by the number of doses – thus, if your child is prescribed 10mg per day of carbamazepine, they will probably take two doses a day, each of 5mg. Some child AEDs are available in liquid form and prescribed doses are likely to be different from those for tablets. Your paediatrician should explain the dosages to you.

Your child should be reviewed by your paediatrician at least once a year, even if their seizures have become stabilised. This is because as they grow, their quantity of medication will need adjusting to match their increased weight.

Generic name	Brand name	Typical daily dose (total)	No. of doses per day	Types of seizures	Common side effects
acetazolamide	Diamox	10-20mg	2	Add-on for tonic-clonic and partial seizures. Sometimes prescribed for atypical absences, tonic and atonic seizures.	Loss of appetite, drowsiness, depression, pins and needles, joint pain, increased urination, thirst, headaches, dizziness, fatigue, irritability.
carbamazepine	Tegretol	10-25mg	2 (3 if in liquid form)	Partial and secondary generalised tonic-clonic seizures, primary generalised seizures.	Skin rash, if allergic. Double vision, unsteadiness and nausea if the starting dose is too high.
clobazam	Frisium	0.25mg	2	Generalised tonic-clonic seizures, partial seizures – one in three children develop tolerance.	Drowsiness, fatigue, depression, irritability.
clonazepam	Rivotril	0.1-0.3mg (under 12 months) 0.3-1mg (age 1-5) 1-2mg (age 5-12)	2-3	Generalised tonic-clonic and partial seizures, absences, myoclonic seizures, Lennox-Gastaut syndrome, infantile spasms, status epilepticus.	Increase in bronchial secretions, fatigue, aggression, hyperactivity, drowsiness. Some children develop tolerance.
ethosuximide	Emeside, Zarontin	15-35mg	2	Absences.	Nausea, drowsiness, headaches.

gabapentin	Neurontin	30-60mg	2-3	Partial seizures where other AEDs proved ineffective.	Drowsiness, dizziness, headaches, fatigue, double vision, unsteadiness.
lamotrigine	Lamictal	0.5-8.0mg if sodium valproate is also prescribed. Otherwise 2-12mg when taken alone or with any other AED.	2	Partial seizures, absences, generalised tonic-clonic seizures, Lennox-Gastaut syndrome.	Skin rash, if allergic or dosage increased too quickly. Drowsiness, double vision, dizziness, headaches, insomnia, tremors, flu-like symptoms. If sodium valproate is also prescribed, there may be tremors.
levetiracetam	Keppra	10-60mg	2	Partial or generalised seizures in children aged four and older.	Dizziness, nausea, sedation, behavioural problems.
nitrazepam	Mogadon	0.5mg	2-3	Infantile spasms.	Confusion, tremors, weak muscles, memory problems.
oxcarbazepine	Trileptal	10-50mg (not licensed for children below the age of six).	2	Generalised tonic-clonic seizures, partial seizures.	Skin rash, if allergic. Double vision, unsteadiness, headaches, nausea, confusion.
phenobarbitone		4-8mg	2	Generalised tonic-clonic and partial seizures, status epilepticus, neonatal seizures.	Drowsiness on starting. Persistent lethargy, sedation and slow mental performance, fatigue, listlessness, depression, rashes, insomnia, irritability, hyperactivity, aggression, impaired memory, moodiness, learning difficulties.

phenytoin	Epanutin	4-8mg	2	Generalised tonic-clonic and partial seizures, status epilepticus.	Skin rash, if allergic. Drowsiness, unsteadiness, slurring if the dose is too high. Prolonged use can cause coarsening of facial features, overgrowth of gums, excess hair growth, acne and anaemia. Shaky or unsteady gait, rapid involuntary eye movements.
primidone	Mysoline	20-30mg	2	Partial and generalised tonic-clonic seizures.	Fatigue, restlessness, psychosis, depression, hyperactivity, irritability.
sodium valproate, sodium valproate modified release	Epilim, Epilim Chrono	20-40mg	2 (once a day for Chrono)	Generalised tonic-clonic and partial seizures, absences.	Short-term hair loss (reversible) on starting. Drowsiness, tremors, weight gain, gastric problems, hyperactivity, behavioural problems.
tiagabine	Gabitril	5-30mg (note: this is not per kilo)	3	Partial seizures where other AEDs proved ineffective.	Dizziness, fatigue, depression, nervousness, tremors, loss of concentration, depression, agitation, anxiety, jerky limbs.
topiramate	Topamax	6-12mg (not licensed for children below the age of two)	2	Partial and generalised seizures, severe myoclonic epilepsy in infancy.	Headaches, drowsiness, dizziness, pins and needles, weight loss, kidney stones. Possible speech disorder or slowed mental performance.
vigabatrin	Sabril	20-100mg, 150mg for infantile spasms	2	Partial seizures resistant to other AEDs, frontline AED for infantile spasms.	Drowsiness, nausea, behaviour/mood swings, visual field defects. Visual field tests should be done every six months.

As with adult AEDs, children need to be carefully weaned on and off any medication. This helps minimise side effects and the possibility of actually triggering seizures.

Administering emergency medication

When children go into status epilepticus it is vital that emergency medication is given quickly. Children who regularly go into status should have a prescription for this. There are two AEDs that can stop continuous seizures – rectal diazepam and buccal midazolam. Professional training is required to give either of these drugs correctly. As a parent, you should automatically be given training once it becomes apparent that status is a regular problem for your child. If your child attends a nursery or school, at least one member of staff there should be trained to administer the medication. Your paediatrician should advise on arranging any training.

Ketogenic diet

The ketogenic diet was developed in the 1920s as a means of helping children with severe epilepsy who don't respond to drug treatment. As more effective epileptic drugs became available, the diet waned in popularity, but interest has grown again in recent years. A number of research studies, the most recent being a controlled trial conducted in 2008 jointly by the Institute of Child Health, Great Ormond Street Hospital and University College London, have demonstrated beyond doubt that the diet can be very beneficial for children with hard-to-control epilepsy.

How it works

The ketogenic diet is a low carbohydrate, low protein and high fat diet that fools the body into thinking it is being starved. Usually when carbohydrates are eaten they are converted into glucose which the body uses as fuel. As the ketogenic diet contains almost no carbohydrates, the body burns fat instead and the liver converts the fat into fatty acids and ketones which the brain uses as its fuel. The production of ketones (called ketosis) has an anticonvulsant effect.

The diet is very strict and requires a major commitment by parents – every single portion of food must be weighed and the correct proportions of each food group calculated. The child has to have the right amount of calories for their age and size but not become overweight from the high fat levels, as well as having an intake of all essential nutrients.

The ketogenic diet usually has a ratio of four parts fat to one part combined protein and carbohydrate. A dietician will produce a suitable eating plan and train you in meal preparation – the ketogenic diet can be adapted for most diets, including religious or ethnic ones, as well as for your child's own food preferences. There are very few side effects, although most children will experience some nausea, tiredness and constipation at first. These usually clear up once the body has adjusted to the diet. Some children will have problems with constipation and vomiting for the whole time they are on the diet. You will be asked to record any changes in your child, such as seizure frequency, and details of their overall wellbeing.

Will it help my child?

The ketogenic diet can be tried on any child aged between one and 16, usually for a minimum of three months. However, there are no guarantees that it will definitely improve your child's epilepsy. Some children show an improvement fairly quickly, while others may need quite a few weeks before any changes show up. For some children, it makes no difference at all. It will be clear within three months if your child is benefiting from the diet or not.

While on the diet, your paediatrician will monitor your child regularly for improvements in their epilepsy, including any changes needed to their AEDs, as well as their overall health. Your child will also have regular EEG tests to measure any on-going epileptical activity in the brain and the paediatrician will ask you to measure and record the level of ketosis in your child. You will be given a simple kit to test either their urine or their blood for ketones and you will need to take this record to every review you have.

Success rate

Roughly 10% of children who try the ketogenic diet become completely seizure-free and may later be able to come off their AEDs. If they stay seizure-fee for two years, then it is possible to discontinue the diet. Around 50% will achieve a moderate to high reduction in the number of overall seizures. However, some may need to stay on the diet longer or try a modified version.

It takes two to three months to be weaned off the diet. During that time the ketogenic ratio will be gradually lowered by the dietician until ketosis can no longer be detected. There is a one in five chance that your child's seizures may return within two years of stopping the diet. If this happens then your child may need to go back on the diet or take AEDs again.

Surgical treatments

Having brain surgery or a vagal nerve stimulator will depend on the type and severity of your child's epilepsy, as well as their age. Your paediatrician will recommend exploring these options if they think your child may benefit from surgery of some sort. Surgical options are discussed in more depth in chapter 3.

Safety issues

Chapter 4 gives detailed information on how to stay safe when you have seizures and this applies to children as much as adults.

Unless your child is severely disabled, he or she should be able to participate safely in most activities. Almost all sports are safe, even swimming, as long as simple precautions are taken. It can be tempting to wrap your child in cotton wool, but if they are not allowed to kick a football around with their friends or join in with playground activities, you risk denting their social life and your child is likely to resent unnecessary restrictions. This could make them more rebellious as they enter their teens. As hard as you may find it, you need to give them as much freedom to participate as possible.

Your child may benefit from some items of safety equipment depending on the type and severity of their seizures. For example, if your child has tonic or atonic seizures (drop attacks), a safety helmet can protect them from head injuries. The help list has details of companies that supply safety aids.

Benefits

If your child has severe disabilities resulting from their epilepsy, they may be entitled to a disability payment benefit to cover the extra costs for care and supervision. The Benefit Enquiry Line can advise you further – call 0800 882 200. Your local social services may also be able to help with grants for special equipment or offer other forms of help – you may qualify for respite care, for example, or to have a carer help out regularly.

Summing Up

Caring for a child with epilepsy can be immensely challenging. It can take time to go through the diagnosis process which can mean spending a lot of time at clinics having your child tested. The paediatrician is also likely to want to see your child at least twice a year to review their progress.

At home you will need to develop routines for giving your child their medication. If you are using the ketogenic diet, you will need to follow this strictly in order to obtain results.

Your child may have extra educational needs as a result of their epilepsy and you will need time and patience to explore all the options available to ensure your child has their schooling needs met.

Teenagers

If you're a teenager and you have epilepsy, read the other chapters for information about seizures, medication and all the other general stuff about epilepsy. This chapter is about the specific things that are relevant to you right now.

Your treatment

Until you reach 16, you'll probably still be seeing a paediatric specialist about your epilepsy. After your 16th birthday, your care will be transferred at some point to a neurologist who treats adults. This may also be the first time you have an opportunity to make your own decisions with the doctor about your treatment. Having more say will help you feel more in control of your epilepsy, so don't be afraid to get involved and ask lots of questions.

If you've had a certain type of epilepsy since you were little, such as absences, you may grow out of this and your doctor will want to discuss stopping your medication and seeing how you go. However, you'll still need to attend follow-up appointments to help check if your seizures have stopped for good or if you need to go back on medication. You'll be growing a lot now too, so your doctor may want to adjust how much medication you take or try you on a different drug designed for adults rather than children.

Telling friends

You probably have mates who've known you for a long time because you go to school together. They'll know about your epilepsy and accept it as part of you, which is great. However, this is a time when you may be changing schools or making new friends outside school because you share interests like music.

Deciding when to tell new friends can be hard. Maybe you're okay with being open about your epilepsy, but maybe you'd rather people got to know you better first before you told them, in case they judge you. And what happens if you decide to wait but then you have a seizure when you're with them? Imagining how you might feel if this happens can help you decide about when you trust a new friend enough to tell them.

How new friends react to you having a seizure can also show you what someone's really like. Hanging out with cool people can make us cool too, but your cool friend isn't really so cool if they start treating you like an idiot or calling you names after you've had a seizure.

Talking to other people your age who have epilepsy can really help as you will have loads in common and you will understand each other's feelings well. There are some great forums on the Internet for teenagers with epilepsy and you might make some new friends! Check out the help list at the back for more information.

Going out

Just because you have epilepsy it doesn't mean that you can't have a good time with your friends. Going to gigs or clubbing is unlikely to give you any problems unless you have photo-sensitive epilepsy (where you react to flashing lights or flickering). If your seizures are stress-related, you'll need to think through the risks about some activities as overexcitement could trigger a seizure. There's no reason why you can't play football or most other sports either. You might want to have a trusted friend with you if you go out – someone who knows what to do if you have a seizure.

Your parents may be overprotective, not wanting you to go out at night in case anything happens to you. You may have to reassure them a lot and show you can be sensible about taking care of yourself.

Drink and drugs

You've probably had discussions about alcohol and drugs in your PSHE class at school, but you need to know extra facts if you have epilepsy as they can increase your risk of having a seizure. Read chapter 4 for information on these risks.

If you're going to try alcohol, go slowly and carefully and test your reactions. It can be really difficult when you're out with your mates and they're all drinking as it can put pressure on you to join in. This could be a time when you have to be really strong-minded about doing your own thing and finding your own safe level to drink at.

The chance of you being around people who take drugs or offer them to you is probably going to be high. This is the time in your life when you're most likely to experiment with them. At some point you'll be making a decision to try drugs or walk away from them. If you do decide to try them, remember that drugs increase your chance of having seizures – that's a very big risk to take. Don't forget drugs are illegal – if you get caught, you could end up with a criminal record and that could damage your chance of training for your dream career.

Relationships

Your PSHE classes at school should cover general issues about relationships, sex and contraception. Dating people, falling in love and experimenting with sex is tricky enough for anyone at your age. When you have epilepsy, you can feel even more insecure. You may have lots of extra questions:

- When should I tell a girlfriend or boyfriend I have epilepsy?
- What if I really like someone but they reject me because of my epilepsy?
- What if I have a seizure on a date or when we're having sex?
- Will my medication cause problems in bed?

You may find it helpful to talk with your epilepsy nurse about these or any other worries you have. Or you could chat online with other teenagers who have epilepsy and find out how they deal with any problems. And remember that older people with epilepsy worry about all these questions too. These are questions you may have to deal with throughout your life because these issues don't ever really go away. You just get a bit wiser about coping!

Studying

If you're still at school, your teachers should be aware of any special needs you have, like needing extra time to do exams or homework. Some kinds of epilepsy medication can make your thoughts feel slow, for example. If you've had a seizure, you may need time off to recuperate – your teachers will understand and will help you catch up on any missed lessons so you don't fall behind.

If you decide to study at college or university, the law protects you from discrimination. This means you can't be refused a place at university because of your epilepsy if you get all the required exam grades at A Level.

As with school, your tutors should be aware of your special needs when it comes to keeping up with the other students. Many colleges assign you a personal tutor in freshers' week – this is someone who you can talk to during your whole course about any educational or personal concerns you may have. If you have a personal tutor, this is the first person you should tell about your epilepsy as they can help coordinate whoever else you think needs to be told.

If you go to a local college or university, you may decide to stay living at home with your family. If you have chosen to study elsewhere, you'll need to register with a doctor on campus if there is a health clinic there or a local GP. Whoever you register with will arrange to have your medical records transferred from your last GP and they should also refer you to a consultant locally who can manage your epilepsy care.

Starting a job

Read chapter 9 for general information on employment and work issues that you need to consider when you have epilepsy. If you decide to leave school and start work instead of going to college, the law protects you from discrimination – you can't be refused a job just because you have epilepsy.

Some jobs will, unfortunately, be closed to you. The Armed Forces are exempt from the Disability Discrimination Act and are unlikely to offer you a position even if your seizures are fully controlled. The various police forces in the UK are becoming increasingly included in the Act, but if you have uncontrolled seizures you are unlikely to pass the fitness test required for joining. Some forces may offer access to civilian jobs such as IT support.

Most other jobs should be open to you. Jobs in which having uncontrolled seizures put you or others at risk – jobs involving working at heights, near water or with fire or chemicals, for example, or if you need to drive or operate dangerous machinery – will be very hard to access unless you can get your seizures under full control. Otherwise, as long as you have any necessary qualifications or suitable experience, you should be employable.

Have a talk with the careers adviser at school or university about your options. They should help you do any research into jobs that interest you, to check you won't be excluded under the law or health and safety rules.

Living away from home

If you're over 16, you might be starting to think about moving out, but your parents may be putting pressure on you to stay. While they know they won't be able to protect you forever, they will want to be very sure that you'll be safe once you become independent.

You'll probably have to agree on compromises such as sharing a flat with others rather than living alone. And your parents will want to be reassured that you will take your medication as usual and stick to your appointments with your doctors. If you are close to one of your brothers or sisters, they may be able to support your arguments for becoming more independent.

Parents can be a bit of a pain at times because they don't always understand you. You're bound to disagree on lots of things but if you can manage to have a sensible chat about the practicalities of moving out – without any arguing or anyone stomping off in a huff – they will feel a lot more comfortable about getting used to the idea of you going, and you'll have proved your maturity to them (This whole discussion may be easier for you all to handle if you've been offered the chance to study elsewhere). Have a chat with your doctor or epilepsy nurse about any practical issues you might need help with if you want to live independently.

Summing Up

Your teenage years are a period of major change as you start growing up and becoming an adult. It can also be a period when you feel vulnerable emotionally and you think people don't really understand you. When you have epilepsy, all these things can seem even more complicated and worrying. However hard it may seem at times, keep the lines of communication open at home with your family. Negotiating the minefield of making new friends and your first relationships will be easier if you can count on your family's support. Your family will also help you as you start moving towards adulthood and becoming independent.

Working Life

Most people with epilepsy are able to work fulltime without any problems. However, not all jobs may be open to you and, depending on your type of epilepsy and how well controlled your seizures are, you will need to take various issues into account.

Making career choices

The only area of work that is completely off-limits to anyone with epilepsy is joining the army, navy or air force, as the Armed Forces are exempt from the Disability Discrimination Act (DDA). The police forces also used to be exempt but are now open, although you may not be able to do active service in a frontline role.

Depending on your seizures, some jobs may or may not be open to you as they are covered by health and safety regulations. This includes any jobs that involve driving (see chapter 5 for information on driving rules) or could put your or other's safety at risk if your seizures are not fully controlled. This could rule out manual occupations that mean you need to work at heights, near water or with fire or chemicals.

If you have set your heart on a particular career, you will need to do some research to find out whether you're going to be able to pursue your dream. If you have developed epilepsy as an adult, you may find you can no longer do your job because of health and safety rules. If this is the case, your employer should move you to another position if possible, or you may decide to retrain.

Jobs involving computers should not present any problems unless you have photo-sensitive epilepsy. Old-style monitors can flicker but the new flat-screen monitors are perfectly safe.

Help finding the right job

Whether you're entering the job market for the first time or planning a career change, you can discuss your options with a disability employment adviser (DEA) at your local JobCentre Plus. The DEA can help you look at any potential restrictions on jobs you are interested in or assist with access to courses if you want to retrain. They can provide much-needed support and advice when it comes to exploring realistic options.

Working shifts

Shift-work can cause problems if you have epilepsy, particularly if you do overnight or late-night shifts. Getting regular sleep is essential to managing your epilepsy and minimising the possibility of seizures. If you have nocturnal epilepsy, shift-work could aggravate your seizures because of the disruption to your body's normal rhythms. Talk to your employer to see if you can change your hours or have more days off in between batches of shifts.

Disclosing your epilepsy

You do not have to tell your employer about your epilepsy but you should consider the consequences of not saying anything. Much will depend on how your epilepsy affects you and whether your job is subject to health and safety regulations.

Disclosure is a tricky issue for many people. Job application forms often ask for information on your health – you could decide to put 'to be discussed at interview' on this part of the form, or even not to say anything until you have had a firm offer for the position. Be aware that if you say nothing and your employer finds out later, you could be in breach of your contract and lose your job if your epilepsy has potentially put others at risk. It may also be useful to ask your GP or neurologist for a letter of support.

Telling your employer means they will have the opportunity to make any adjustments in the workplace to enable you to work without any problems. At some point you may also have to deal with telling immediate colleagues, particularly if your seizures are uncontrolled. Telling your workmates means you can explain what they can do to help you if you have a seizure at work. Talking about your epilepsy before they see you have a seizure may make you feel more in control of the disclosure process.

Discrimination in the workplace

The DDA covers your right to equality in the workplace, taking into account the job restrictions mentioned above. You cannot be refused a position simply because you have epilepsy. If there are minor health and safety issues (i.e. those that do not mean your or others' safety will be compromised), your employer should make 'reasonable adjustments' to enable you to perform your duties. This could mean changing your computer monitor or giving you time off to recuperate from a seizure or to attend medical appointments. If your seizures change or worsen, reasonable adjustments could also mean offering you a different position or changing your hours. Sometimes such changes need only be temporary.

Discrimination can sometimes be hard to prove but if you think you have been discriminated against at work because of your epilepsy, you may have grounds to bring a case. Consult your union rep if you have one. Chapter 10 offers further advice.

Insurance and pensions

Under the Health and Safety at Work Act, employers have to have insurance for their staff. The insurance provides compensation if you have an accident at work or are injured. If you haven't disclosed your epilepsy to your employer, you may not be covered if anything happens to you.

You are entitled to the same pension rights as your colleagues and you cannot be excluded from a company pension scheme because you have epilepsy. However, your epilepsy may be taken into account if you take out a private pension. You may also have to pay higher premiums if you want your policy to include an option for early retirement on health grounds because of the risk of SUDEP. You should consult a qualified financial adviser if you are considering a private pension scheme.

Working Tax Credit

You may be eligible for Working Tax Credit (WTC) which has a disability element. The relevant part is the Disadvantage Test – if ‘at least once a year during waking hours you are in a coma or have a fit in which you lose consciousness’ and you also fulfil the basic conditions of eligibility for WTC, you should make a claim. You can call the Tax Office for a claim pack on 0345 300 3900. The Tax Office can also help you if you need assistance filling the claim form in. Claims are generally backdated to the date of application but you may qualify to have it backdated an additional three months.

Access to Work

If you need help in the workplace as a result of having epilepsy, such as having equipment adapted or needing help getting to and from work if you have problems using public transport, you may qualify for assistance under the Access to Work scheme. The disability employment adviser at your local JobCentre Plus can advise you on your eligibility for assistance.

Self-employment

Working for yourself can be a practical option for many people with epilepsy. The type of work you decide to do will depend on your experience, skills, interests and whether you can find a niche in the market for your services or products. This is a particularly good option if you have a qualified skill in a service like accounting or translation as these are jobs you can do from home that have very low overheads.

Advantages

- Less stressful – no commuting, being bossed around or working to other people's deadlines.
- Flexibility – you can choose your hours which is very useful if your seizures are active and you need to take time out to recuperate or for hospital appointments.
- Control – you have total control over what you do, how you do it and when.
- Satisfaction – many self-employed people say that working for themselves is more satisfying, even if they earn less than when they were an employee.

Disadvantages

- Isolation – no workplace camaraderie.
- Patience – it can take time to build up a business.
- Stress – unless you take on staff, you have to do everything (bookkeeping, admin, project management, etc) which can be very stressful.

If you decide to look into self-employment, talk to your local Business Link or Chamber of Commerce, both of which are experienced in helping people start small businesses and can be found in the Yellow Pages. They can offer plenty of advice and often run free courses that cover issues such as tax, invoicing, bookkeeping and trading standards.

Summing Up

Unless your seizures are very severe, you should be able to work. Some jobs are restricted on health and safety grounds but otherwise you cannot legally be refused a position just because you have epilepsy. Your employer should make any necessary reasonable adjustments so you can carry out your duties on an equal basis. You will need to consider the issue of telling your boss or colleagues but you are not obliged to. Self-employment can be a solution to issues such as the problem of travelling to work or needing flexible hours to accommodate your health needs.

Rights and Welfare Benefits

Disability Discrimination Act

The Disability Discrimination Act (DDA) applies to people with epilepsy. It means you cannot be treated less fairly by employers, educational establishments, landlords or those who provide goods or services to you just because you have epilepsy, and it makes no difference if your seizures are fully controlled with AEDs.

Employers and businesses must make 'reasonable adjustments' under the act to ensure you are treated fairly. For example, a college would need to allow you extra time to complete your essays if you've missed lectures as a result of having seizures. If they refuse to make reasonable adjustments for you, you may have grounds to bring a case against them for discrimination.

There are some exceptions under the act. The Armed Forces are exempt and some other jobs could be closed to you because your seizures would put you or others at risk in the course of your work duties (see chapter 9). You cannot say someone refused to make a reasonable adjustment if the adjustment would in practice be unreasonable, such as expecting a disco not to have strobe lights.

Breaching the DDA is not a criminal offence. This means that any cases of discrimination within the terms of the act are being tested on a case-by-case basis in the civil courts. If you think you have been discriminated against because of your epilepsy, you should take legal advice to see if you have grounds for a case. The Equality and Human Rights Commission is the government-funded body that oversees implementation of the act and can advise you. Alternatively, you could consult the Citizens Advice Bureau or a lawyer who specialises in discrimination. If it's a workplace issue and you have union membership, consult your union rep first.

Prescriptions

If you have epilepsy, you are entitled to free prescriptions on the NHS. This right covers not just free medication for your epilepsy but any medication for any other condition that your doctor or consultant may prescribe for you.

Claiming exemption charges is very easy. Ask your GP surgery to give you a copy of Form FP92A. Fill in the form and ask your GP or consultant to counter-sign it to confirm your entitlement, then return it to the address given on the form. You can also get the form from a hospital or some pharmacies. Processing the application takes around a month, so don't delay in completing your application.

Your exemption certificate will be sent to you by post. It looks like a credit card and contains your name, certificate number and validity period. Medical Exemption Certificates (Medex) are usually valid for five years. You may be sent a reminder by post that your certificate needs to be renewed but not necessarily – it is your responsibility to get it renewed. Make sure you collect a renewal form at least one month before your current certificate expires.

Benefits

The UK benefits system is very complex. Benefits are mostly means-tested – in other words, how much money you receive will depend on whether you live with anyone else and how much joint income you have. Non-means-tested benefits can be applied for regardless of how much income you or others in your household have. This section will only look at disability benefits as epilepsy is legally classed as a disability.

Claim forms for all state benefits can be collected from JobCentre Plus, downloaded from the JobCentre Plus website or you can start a claim by telephone. Claim forms can be very long, sometimes more than 50 pages. If you feel confident enough to complete the form yourself, take a photocopy of it before you return it so you have your own record. You can access free, independent, professional advice and assistance with making a claim from any Citizens Advice Bureau or Welfare Rights Office (these are usually run by your local council). If you have a local disability charity in your area, they may be able to help you complete a claim too.

Benefits claims may be refused when you apply, but you are entitled to ask for a formal review of your application. You can also appeal if your claim is still refused. This may take several months and you will probably have to attend the appeal tribunal, which should be held locally to you. Using a professional adviser to make your initial claim can increase your chance of being awarded benefits quickly.

If you are eligible for some of the following benefits, you may also be entitled to help with Housing Benefit, Council Tax Benefit and Pension or Working Tax Credit.

Disability Living Allowance

Disability Living Allowance (DLA) is a non-means-tested benefit and has two components, care and mobility, which are intended to help towards the extra costs associated with living with a disability. You can be working and still eligible to make a claim.

If you are awarded DLA, you can decide how you spend it. You could use it to buy in professional care at home to help with some tasks or it could help cover the cost of taxis if you need to get to places not served by public transport.

If you apply for DLA, only one criterion determines your eligibility – if you have uncontrolled epileptic seizures and do not have auras (although this is not stated on the application form, but is a legal ruling made by the House of Lords). This is because it is assumed that if you have a warning, you have time to make yourself safe before the seizure starts and are therefore not endangered. The frequency of your seizures should not be taken into account. You will not be awarded DLA if you have auras.

Employment and Support Allowance

Employment and Support Allowance (ESA) replaced Incapacity Benefit at the end of 2008 and you may be able to claim this if your seizures affect your ability to work. The claim criteria are rather complex as ESA is part means-tested and part non-means-tested. ESA is intended to provide temporary financial relief with the aim of you being able to return to work at some point, although you may still be eligible if your epilepsy is so severe that you are not expected to return to work. Note that if you have been in receipt of Incapacity Benefit since before 27 October 2008, you will continue to receive it.

You may be eligible to claim ESA if:

- Your Statutory Sick Pay has ended or you cannot get it.
- You are self-employed or unemployed.
- You were receiving Statutory Maternity Pay but have not returned to work because your epilepsy affects your ability to work.
- You are under state pension age.

You must also either:

- Have seizures that affect your ability to work for at least four days in a row (including weekends and public holidays).
- Be unable to work for two or more days out of seven consecutive days.
- Be getting special medical treatment.

You will have to undergo a Work Capability Assessment (WCA) if you apply for ESA. This is a medical assessment of how your epilepsy affects your ability to work and aims to identify work you can do and what support in the workplace you may need to help you return to work. An assessment rate of ESA is paid during the first 13 weeks while your claim is examined and you have the WCA test. After that you will be placed in one of two groups. Benefit rates become higher at this stage.

- 1. Work Related Activity Group: you will have work-focused interviews with an adviser and be helped back to work.
- 2. Support Group: you will be placed in this group if your epilepsy is so severe you cannot be expected to work.

At time of writing, ESA is so new that independent benefits experts say it is unclear how successful it will be in helping people return to work and ensuring that those people too ill to work will get the financial help they need.

Attendance Allowance

If you are over 65 and have a disability that is so severe you need help to look after yourself, you may be able to claim Attendance Allowance (AA) (under-65s should apply for Disability Living Allowance). AA is not means-tested and you do not usually need to have a medical examination.

Community Care Grant

This one-off payment is usually paid if you are in receipt of certain benefits and need financial help to live in the community, such as coming out of residential care to live independently or to remain in your home instead of going into hospital. You don't have to pay it back. Ask JobCentre Plus for details.

Other benefits

Blue Badge parking scheme

Even if you can't drive because of your epilepsy, you may still qualify for a Blue Badge permit if you receive the higher rate of the Disability Living Allowance Mobility Component and have trouble using public transport or walking because of your seizures. You and your driver can use the Blue Badge to park when you need to be out and about. Apply to your Local Authority (LA) for details.

Disabled Students Allowance

This is paid on top of your student loan and does not have to be repaid. The allowance is to cover the extra costs of being disabled while at university or college so that you can pursue your studies on an equal basis with other students. You can use it to buy special equipment, pay for additional travel costs or towards a carer if you need assistance. Ask your LA for details in the first instance.

LA grants

LAs offer various grants for the disabled, mostly for having your home adapted to help you live independently. Some are means-tested and you usually need to be assessed by social services. These grants include the Disabled Facilities Grant, Direct Payments and the Independent Living Fund. Criteria for eligibility vary. Contact your LA for further information.

Summing Up

The law protects you from discrimination on the grounds of disability if you have epilepsy and ensures you have the right to equal treatment. In addition, your epilepsy entitles you to free prescriptions and you may also be eligible for some state welfare or LA benefits. Take advantage of these – prescriptions are expensive while a successful claim for benefits could ease your financial situation further.

Help List

Epilepsy support organisations

Brainwave – The Irish Epilepsy Association

249 Crumlin Road, Crumlin, Dublin 12

Tel: 01 455 7500

www.epilepsy.ie

Information, education, support, advocacy and training for people with epilepsy in the Republic of Ireland.

The Daisy Garland

2 Stoyle House, 7 South Street, Totnes TQ9 5DZ

Tel: 01803 847 999

www.thedaisygarland.org.uk

Support, advice and information on improving the quality of life for children with hard-to-control epilepsy plus developmental delay.

Epilepsy Action (also known as the British Epilepsy Association)

New Anstey House, Gate Way Drive, Yeadon, Leeds, LS19 7XY
Tel: 0808 800 5050 (helpline)

www.epilepsy.org.uk

A national charity that provides support and advice, campaigns to raise awareness of epilepsy, provides Sapphire Nurses for epilepsy clinics and fundraises for research into epilepsy. There are a number of regional branches. The website has a forum (www.forum4e.com) where people with epilepsy and their carers can chat to each other for support and advice.

Epilepsy Bereaved

PO Box 112, Wantage, Oxon, OX12 8XT
Tel: 01235 772 850

info@epilepsybereaved.org.uk

www.sudep.org
This charity offers bereavement support for anyone who has been affected by SUDEP and undertakes research into the causes of SUDEP.

Epilepsy Research UK

PO Box 3004, London, W4 4XT

Tel: 020 8995 4781

www.epilepsyresearch.org.uk

Promotes and supports scientific and medical research into epilepsy.

Epilepsy Scotland

48 Govan Road, Glasgow, G51 1JL

Tel: 0808 800 2200 (helpline)

www.epilepsyscotland.org.uk

Information, campaigns, training, support and advocacy throughout Scotland.

Epilepsy Society

Chesham Lane, Chalfont St Peter, Bucks, SL9 0RJ

Tel: 01494 601 300 (helpline)

www.epilepsysociety.org.uk

A national charity that provides support and advice, campaigns to raise awareness and fundraises for research into epilepsy. It also runs an important residential centre for people with very severe epilepsy who need permanent expert care. The website has a forum (www.epilepsysociety.org.uk/forum) where people with epilepsy and their carers can chat to each other for support and advice.

Epilepsy Wales

Bradbury House, 23 Salisbury Road, Wrexham, LL13 7AS

Tel: 0800 228 9016

www.epilepsy-wales.co.uk

This organisation provides information, support and training for people in Wales who have epilepsy, their families and carers.

FABLE

Lower Ground Floor, 305 Glossop Road, Sheffield, S10 2HL

Tel: 0800 521 629 (helpline)

www.fable.org.uk

Self-help support, advice and advocacy for patients and their families considering VNS therapy.

Joint Epilepsy Council (JEC)

PO Box 186, Leeds, LS20 8WY
Tel: 01943 871852

www.jointepilepsycouncil.org.uk

This umbrella organisation represents 26 epilepsy organisations in the UK and Ireland (contact details for these are on the website and include many regional groups). Its two main aims are to improve the standards of and access to health, education and social care services for people with epilepsy and their carers, and to increase awareness of epilepsy among politicians, civil servants, service providers and the general public.

Matthew's Friends

St Piers Lane, Lingfield, Surrey, RH7 6PW

Tel: 01342 836757

www.matthewsfriends.org

Support and advice for parents who have an epileptic child on the ketogenic diet.

Support Dogs

21 Jessops Riverside, Brightside Lane, Sheffield, S9 2RX

Tel: 0114 261 7800

www.support-dogs.org.uk

Support Dogs trains seizure alert dogs for people with severe epilepsy.

UK Epilepsy and Pregnancy Register

www.epilepsyandpregnancy.co.uk

Comprehensive advice and information on all aspects of pregnancy for women with epilepsy.

VNS Therapy

www.vnstherapy.com

Website of Cyberonics, the company that makes VNS devices. Lots of useful information for patients and their families.

Medication aids

The following companies all sell devices for organising your tablets if you are on medication.

Chester Care (part of Homecraft Rolyan)

Nunn Brook Road, Huthwaite, Sutton in Ashfield, Notts, NG17 2HU

Tel: 08444 124330

www.homecraft-rolyan.com

PivoTell Ltd

PO Box 108, Saffron Walden, CB11 4WX

Tel: 01799 550 979

www.pivotell.co.uk

Tabtime Ltd

41 Park Lane, Sandbach, Cheshire, CW11 1EN

Tel: 01270 767 207

www.tabtime.com

W + W Medsystems

Unit B1, Crosland Road Industrial Estate, Netherton, Huddersfield, HD4 7DQ

Tel: 01484 667 822

www.wwmed.co.uk

Safety and disability aids

Alert It

Atherstone House, Desford, Leicester LE9 9FE

Tel: 0845 217 9952

www.alert-it.co.uk/Epilepsy

Sells bed alarms for people who have nocturnal seizures.

Disabled Living Foundation

380-384 Harrow Road, London, W9 2HU

Tel: 0845 130 9177

www.dlf.org.uk

Advice, support and direct access to suppliers of a variety of equipment to help you live independently.

Easylink UK

3 Melbourne House, Corby Gate Business Park, Priors Haw Road, Corby, Northants, NN17 5JG

Tel: 01536 264 869

www.easylinkuk.co.uk

Sells epilepsy alarms and monitors of various types.

Genie Care

Unit T6, Rudford Industrial Estate, Ford, Littlehampton, West Sussex, BN18 OBF

Tel: 01903 733377

www.geniecare.com

Sells padded bed sides for people with nocturnal seizures

The Helpful Hand

Tel: 01625 424438/617857

www.thehelpfulhand.co.uk

Sells anti-suffocation pillows and other disability equipment

RADAR Keys

12 City Forum, 250 City Road, London, EC1V 8AF

Tel: 020 7250 3222

www.radar-shop.org.uk

Radar keys may also be available from local disability charities.

Sleep Safe

Avondale House, 70 Tarvin Road, Littleton, Chester, CH3 7DF

Tel: 07092 255916

www.sleep-safe.co.uk

Sells anti-suffocation pillows.

Medical ID jewellery and devices

CramAlert

www.cramalert.co.uk

MedicAlert

327-329 Witan Court, Upper 4th Street, ,ilton Keynes MK9 1EH

Tel: 0800 581 420

www.medicalert.org.uk

Meditag

37 Northampton Street, Hockley, Birmingham, B18 6DU

Tel: 0121 212 3636

www.hoopers.org/meditag.asp

SOS Talisman

21 Grays Corner, Ley Street, Ilford, Essex, IG2 7RQ

Tel: 020 8554 5579

www.sostalisman.co.uk

Universal Medical ID

PO Box 1099, Bedford, MK42 7XR

Tel: 0800 055 6504

www.universalmedicalid.com/uk

UTAG

Unit 7, Majestic Road, Nursling Industrial Estate, Southampton, SO16 0YT

Tel: 0845 872 3202

www.utagice.com

Government-run sites

DirectGov

www.direct.gov.uk

A one-stop-shop website where you can find links to departments and government agencies that you may need to deal with.

Driver Vehicle and Licensing Agency (DVLA)

DVLA, Swansea, SA6 7JL

Tel: 0300 123 0784

www.dvla.gov.uk

Driver and Vehicle Agency Northern Ireland

Tel: 0028 7034 1398

www.dvlni.gov.uk

As well as the place to resolve driving licence issues, you can also apply for a SmartPass here for concessionary travel.

Equality and Human Rights Commission

Tel: 0800 444 205

www.equalityhumanrights.com

The EHRC is responsible for overseeing the Disability Discrimination Act (DDA). If you think you may have been discriminated against because of your epilepsy, call the helpline for advice. You can order a copy of the DDA from the Commission or download it from the website.

European Health Insurance Card (EHIC)

Tel: 0845 605 0707

www.ehic.org.uk

An EHIC entitles you to free or reduced-cost medical treatment while you are visiting Europe. You can apply for one online, by phone or by post.

JobCentre Plus

Tel: 0800 055 6688 (benefits helpline)

www.jobcentreplus.gov.uk

JobCentre Plus should be your first port of call for benefit applications, consultation with a disability employment adviser and information on the Access to Work scheme.

National Institute for Health and Clinical Excellence (NICE)

MidCity Place, 71 High Holborn, London, WC1V 6NA

Tel: 0845 003 7780

www.nice.org.uk

Sets guidelines and standards for all kinds of medical treatments, including epilepsy. The Guideline for Epilepsy can be downloaded from www.nice.org.uk/CG020 or contact NICE for a printed version.

Yellow Card scheme

Tel: 0808 100 3352.

www.yellowcard.gov.uk

For reporting side effects of drugs.

Other useful organisations

DIAL UK

St Catherine's, Tickhill Road, Doncaster, DN4 8QN

Tel: 01302 310123

www.dialuk.info

A national umbrella organisation of disability charities. Dial has an extensive network of local branches and can provide advice on welfare benefits, mobility, independent living and many other aspects on disability. Some local branches sell RADAR keys for disabled toilets.

Frank

Tel: 0800 77 66 00

www.talktofrank.com

Confidential advice and information on all kinds of recreational drugs. Aimed at young people.

Travel

Civil Aviation Authority

CAA House, 45-59 Kingsway, London, WC2B 6TE
Tel: 020 7379 7311

www.caa.co.uk

Can advise on your fitness to hold a pilot's licence.

Community Transport Association (CTA)

Highbank, Halton Street, Hyde, Cheshire, SK14 2NY

Tel: 0161 351 1475

www.ctauk.org

The CTA has information on local charitable organisations that can provide transportation if you need assistance.

Disabled Persons Railcard

PO Box 11631, Laurencekirk, AB30 9AA
Tel: 0845 605 0525

www.disabledpersons-railcard.co.uk

Visit the website for information on obtaining a railcard.

Yellow Cross

PO Box 448, Farnham, Surrey, GU9 8ZU

Tel: 01252 820321

www.yellowcross.co.uk

Yellow Cross sells medical travel kits that are particularly suitable if you are travelling abroad.

Education

Advisory Centre for Education (ACE)

United House, North Road, London N7 9DP

Tel: 0808 800 5793

www.ace-ed.org.uk

Independent advice and support for those needing help negotiating the special educational needs system.

Book List

Both Epilepsy Action and the National Society for Epilepsy produce an extensive range of specialist pamphlets, booklets, factsheets, CDs and DVDs on all aspects of epilepsy. Some of these can be downloaded from their websites while others can be ordered free or for a small charge. The following books may be useful for more in-depth information.

Epilepsy: A Practical Guide (Resource Materials for Teachers)

By Mike Johnson and Gill Parkinson, David Fulton Publishers, UK, 2002, £21.99.

Covering every aspect of the UK education system from what epilepsy is through to learning difficulties and the special educational needs system. Despite the title, this book is very useful for parents as well as education professionals who come into contact with epileptic children.

Epilepsy and Your Child

By Dr Richard Appleton, Brian Chappell and Margaret Beirne, Class Publishing, Revised Edition, London, 2004, £14.99.

A very comprehensive and easy-to-read guide to epilepsy in childhood, with detailed information on all kinds of questions you may not have thought of.

Epilepsy the Natural Way

By Fiona Marshall, Vega Books, 2002.

The definitive guide to a huge range of complementary therapies for treating epilepsy, either without medication or in combination with AEDs.

Glossary

Add-on treatment

Use of a secondary drug to improve seizure control.

Adjunctive therapy

Use of two or more drugs to improve seizure control.

AEDs

Anti-epileptic drugs. This is the common term for prescription medications used to control epileptic seizures.

Ambulatory EEG

See also EEG. The ambulatory version of this standard test usually takes 24 hours and allows you to be fully mobile, including being at home or engaging in most usual activities.

Anti-convulsant

Drug used to control seizures.

Aura

Technically, an aura is a simple partial seizure, but it is often a warning sign that you are about to have a complex partial or generalised seizure. The aura may be as simple as feeling dizzy or 'odd' or may involve fluttery feelings in the tummy or nausea.

Benign rolandic epilepsy

One in five children with epilepsy have BRE. It is characterised by partial temporal lobe seizures, often after waking, accompanied by twitching. BRE responds very well to medication and most children will grow out of it by puberty.

Buccal midazolam

An emergency medication to prevent status epilepticus. It is given by mouth and needs to be administered by a trained person.

Childhood absence seizures

This syndrome is very common, usually beginning in mid-childhood and characterised by absences where the child appears to be daydreaming or staring into space. It is easily diagnosed, responds well to medication and most children grow out of it during adolescence.

Combination therapy

Use of at least two drugs to improve seizure control.

Déjà vu

A common feature of temporal lobe epilepsy where you have the feeling you have done something or have been somewhere before. The opposite is jamais vu, where you have the sensation that what you are seeing, or where you are, is unknown to you when it is in fact very familiar.

Dual therapy

Use of a secondary drug to improve seizure control.

EEG

Electroencephalogram – a standard diagnostic test that measures and records epileptical activity in the brain.

Lennox-Gastaut syndrome

One of the most severe childhood epilepsies, L-G is characterised by multiple seizure types that do not respond well to drug treatment and progressive mental deterioration. L-G children do not often live to see adulthood.

Monotherapy

Use of a single drug to control seizures.

Neurologist

A specialist in medical conditions that affect the nervous system including the brain. Not all neurologists specialise in epilepsy.

Parallel imports

You may hear this term used in connection with your AEDs. It refers to medication that is imported into the UK, usually from another EU country. Although the active ingredient of the generic drug will be identical, the 'filler' ingredients may be different and there is a possibility this could affect your seizures. Also, the leaflet may be in a foreign language and the tablets may be a different colour or size than you are used to.

Polytherapy

Use of additional drugs to improve seizure control.

Post-ictal

A term used to describe the recovery phase after a seizure.

Protocol

This is the official name for a written treatment plan for your epilepsy. Protocols are usually drawn up where your epilepsy is known to have additional complications, such as if you regularly go into status epilepticus. The protocol will cover instructions for when to administer medication or to call for emergency help.

Rectal diazepam

An emergency medication to prevent status epilepticus. It is administered by a trained person via the patient's rectum (up the bottom).

Seizure threshold

This is your own individual level of resistance to having seizures. Someone with a high threshold may never have a single seizure in their lifetime while someone with a lower threshold may suddenly develop epilepsy in later life if something happens to tip them over the edge of their threshold, such as a head injury.

Tertiary service

A top-tier specialist level of patient care. This usually involves being treated at a specialist centre for that condition (sometimes called a centre of excellence).

Trigger

Something that causes a seizure. Many people with epilepsy have common triggers such as tiredness, alcohol, stress or flashing lights (for the 5% who have photo-sensitive epilepsy), but many people do not have triggers at all. A trigger could be anything – over-exercising to the point of exhaustion or hormonal fluctuations, for example – and may be unusual and quite specific to that individual.

Video telemetry

An EEG in which you are videoed during the test so the technician can observe your movements for typical physical clues to epilepsy.

Need – 2 – Know

Need - 2 - Know

Other Large Print Titles Include ...

Allergies A Parent's Guide
ISBN 978-1-86144-160-7 £12.99

Autism A Parent's Guide
ISBN 978-1-86144-165-2 £12.99

Drugs A Parent's Guide
ISBN 978-1-86144-136-2 £12.99

Dyslexia A Parent's Guide
ISBN 978-1-86144-138-6 £12.99

Bullying A Parent's Guide
ISBN 978-1-86144-137-9 £12.99

Epilepsy The Essential Guide
ISBN 978-1-86144-152-2 £12.99

Teenage Pregnancy The Essential Guide
ISBN 978-1-86144-139-3 £12.99

Gap Years The Essential Guide
ISBN 978-1-86144-169-0 £12.99

How to Pass Exams A Parent's Guide
ISBN 978-1-86144-140-9 £12.99

Child Obesity A Parent's Guide
ISBN 978-1-86144-141-6 £12.99

Applying for a Job The Essential Guide
ISBN 978-1-86144-180-5 £12.99

ADHD The Essential Guide
ISBN 978-1-86144-145-4 £12.99

Student Cookbook – Healthy Eating
The Essential Guide
ISBN 978-1-86144-146-1 £12.99

Stress The Essential Guide
ISBN 978-1-86144-147-8 £12.99

Your First Pregnancy The Essential Guide
ISBN 978-1-86144-158-4 £12.99

Special Educational Needs A Parent's Guide
ISBN 978-1-86144-149-2 £12.99

The Pill An Essential Guide
ISBN 978-1-86144-150-8 £12.99

University A Survival Guide
ISBN 978-1-86144-153-9 £12.99

Visit **www.need2knowbooks.co.uk** for the full range. To order our titles call **01733 898103**, email **sales@n2kbooks.com** or visit the website. Selected ebooks available online.

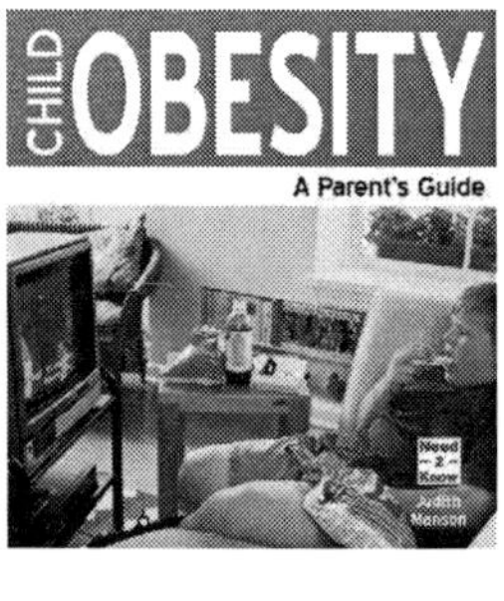

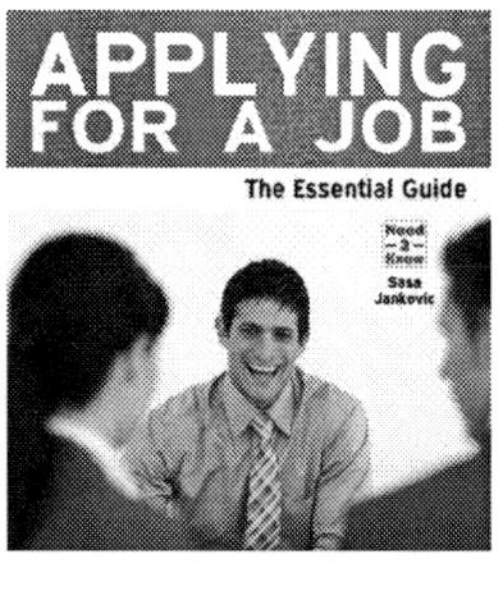

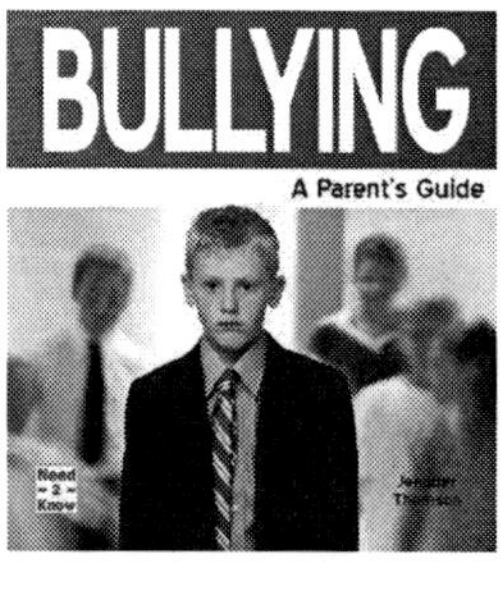

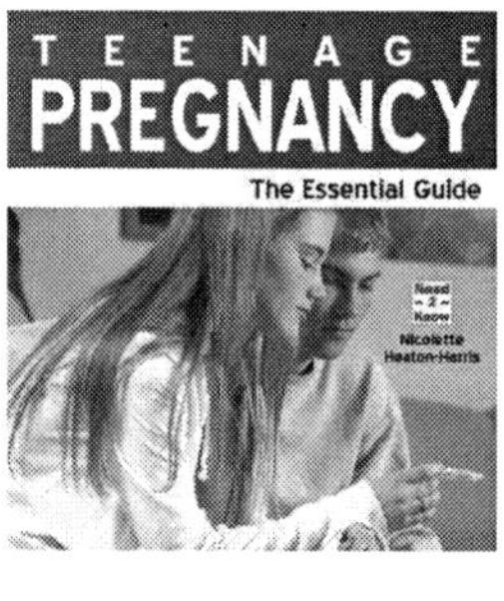

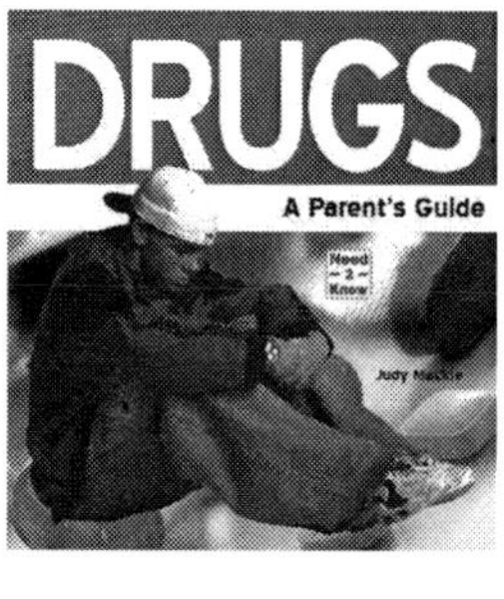

Need - 2 - Know, Remus House, Coltsfoot Drive, Peterborough, PE2 9BF